ANCIENT WAY TO KEEP FIT

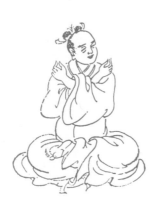

EXERCISES ILLUSTRATED:

ANCIENT WAY TO KEEP FIT

COMPILED BY

ZONG WU • LI MAO

TRANSLATED BY

SONG LUZENG
LIU BEIJIAN
LIU ZHENKAI

PAINTINGS BY

ZHANG KE REN

FOREWORD BY

KUMAR FRANTZIS

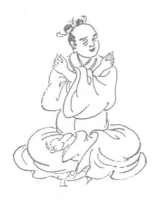

SHELTER

SHELTER PUBLICATIONS INC
BOLINAS CALIFORNIA USA

Distributed in the United States and Canada by
Publishers Group West, Berkeley, California

**Library of Congress
Cataloging in Publication Data**

Chung-kuo tai yang sheng t'u p'u. English: Ancient way to keep fit/
    compiled by Zong Wu, Li Mao: translated by Song Luzeng,
    Liu Beijian, Liu Zhenkai.
    p.   cm.
    Published in Hong Kong in 1990 in both Chinese and English
    (under title: Exercises Illustrated)—Publisher's note.
    ISBN 0-936070-14-5: $18.95
    1. Ch'i kung.   I. Zong Wu.   II. Li Mao.   III. Title
    IV Title: Exercises illustrated.
    RA 781.8.C4913   1992
    613.7'148—dc20   92-81013
                                                                     CIP

First American printing 1992
8 7 6 5 4 3 — 05 04 03 02 01 00
(Lowest digits indicate number and year of latest printing)
Printed in Korea

Additional copies of this book may be purchased at your local bookstore, or by sending $18.95 plus $3.95 shipping/handling to:

**Shelter Publications, Inc.
P. O. Box 279
Bolinas, California 94924 USA
www.shelterpub.com**

Note to the Reader: Be careful with many of the exercises and positions shown in this book, especially if you have not exercised for a while. If you have (or have had) any health problems, especially lower back problems, consult with your physician before attempting any of these exercises. Proceed slowly. If you feel any pain, stop and find an easier position that does not cause pain.

> *Know when to stop
> And you will meet with no danger.*
> –Lao Tzu/Tao Te Ching
> translated by D. C. Lau

Publisher's Note

We are proud to present this unique book on Taoist exercise. It was compiled, written and illustrated in mainland China, and published in Hong Kong in 1990 in both Chinese and English.

Ancient Way to Keep Fit is an intriguing (and aesthetic) introduction to traditional Chinese health practices, most notably the art of *Chi Gung*. Chi Gung (or *Qigong*) is a Chinese word for Taoist exercises that balance and strengthen the flow of *chi* (or *qi),* the life force, the connecting link between body, mind, and spirit.

There are 30 sets of exercises in this book, all taken from classical Chinese sources. Please note that the instructions in this book alone will not provide you with a very deep understanding of the subtle and powerful forces at work in Chi Gung. But they, along with the drawings, will give you a feeling of the movement, the look, and the spirit of these "internal martial arts" exercises. You are encouraged to select one or two sets to practice, according to your fitness level. When practicing, if you feel something happening, or you sense something *could* happen, and wish to proceed, seek out an experienced teacher—the best way to learn—or more detailed books on the subject.

In this American edition, we have not altered the original English of the text, nor have we attempted to rewrite the instructions. We have limited our changes to a few minor ones, some warnings next to certain positions, and a glossary of unfamiliar words (on pp. 210–211). We felt that to westernize the text would dilute the distinctive Chinese flavor of the language and to attempt to rewrite the instructions for these subtle movements would be highly complex. It is our hope that readers will appreciate, as did we, a more direct communication with present-day China than an edited version would provide.

*   *   *

There was a mass revival of Chi Gung in China in the '70s and '80s, and classes are now becoming more widely available in this country. Taoist exercise seems to appear at a fortuitous time on the American scene. Most Americans, it turns out, are not inclined to follow the intense athletic training regimens popularized over the past two decades, and this gentle and calm—yet effective —approach to increased energy and more vibrant health could be what many people have been looking for.

The Foreword is written by Kumar Frantzis, an American fluent in both Chinese and Japanese, with over 30 years experience in martial arts, healing and meditation, including 10 years study in China. Frantzis was formerly a tournament Karate champion in Japan and has black belts in Karate, Aikido, Judo and Ju-jitsu. In 1981, he became the first Westerner certified by the People's Republic of China to teach the complete system of Tai Chi. He is also a lineage disciple of Liu Hung Chieh of Beijing in Wu style Tai Chi and Pa Kua.

> *Hold fast to the way of antiquity*
> *In order to keep in control the realm of today*
> – Tao Te Ching

Contents

Foreword

The elegant Oriental watercolors in this book represent a series of ancient Chinese exercises known as Chi Gung. Chi Gung systems have been recognized in China for over 4000 years for their ability to eliminate illness, heal injury, and mitigate (if not reverse) many of the unwanted conditions brought on by aging. Chi Gung practice is also noted for being the secret source of the internal power of martial arts masters, as well as of the great meditation masters and mystics.

What Is Chi?

Chinese medicine views the individual human being as one interconnected and inseparable whole of body, mind, and spirit, and it treats illness from this point of view. That which connects the whole together is the *chi*. In Chinese thought, chi is the life force energy that powers the "machine" of the body. Chi is the power source that enables your eyes to see, your mouth to taste, your muscles to move, your internal organs and glands to function, and your mind to think. Chi is the human equivalent of the electricity that makes a television work: without electricity to drive it, a television becomes merely a useless shell filled with silicon chips and wiring. In the same way, without chi, the body and its organs are useless.

What Is Chi Gung?

Chi Gung is the ancient science that imparts how individuals can, through their own efforts, balance and strengthen their own chi, even as the body ages. Whereas the body's "hardware" is genetically programmed to degenerate with age, the chi, properly cultivated, can become increasingly stronger during one's lifetime and counteract the undesirable affects of aging. Chi Gung exercises promote a longevity in which people can be as alive, aware, and functional at the end of their lives as they were in youth. These exercises are as valuable – and as accessible – to a senior citizen recovering from a heart attack as they are to a young person or to a competitive athlete.

The Background of Chi Gung

There are five major branches of Chi Gung in China: Taoist, Buddhist, medical, martial arts, and Confucian. The exercises depicted in this book are drawn from the first four. The original Chi Gung was Taoist, which was the source for the others. The Taoist form created Chinese medicine over 4000 years ago, discovering the points and meridian lines of acupuncture and the medicinal uses of thousands of herbs.

Taoist Chi Gung equally emphasizes cultivating physical vitality and developing spirit or consciousness through meditation. It seeks long life with vibrant health into old age, as well as a living spiritual awareness that manifests daily here and now, not in an afterlife. In contrast, Buddhist Chi Gung focuses more on the health of the soul than that of the body.

The other three branches of Chi Gung borrowed techniques from both the Taoists and Buddhists, and recombined them for specific purposes. For example, the Confucians stress applying Chi Gung to intellectual or aesthetic practices, such as painting or calligraphy; medical Chi Gung utilizes chi to cure disease, relieve pain, heal injuries, and maintain ongoing wellness; martial arts Chi Gung seeks to create exceptional physical abilities and psychic awareness.

How Chi Gung Is Practiced

All Chi Gung exercises are performed in a relaxed, gentle fashion that does not cause shock to the body. All stretches must be done to only 70 percent of capacity, not 100 percent. Chi Gung exercises are the most effective and sophisticated low-impact exercises that have ever existed. Chi Gung does not build dynamic muscles; rather, it uses breathing, stretching, movement, and visualization to develop chi, a strong, functional body, and a calm and relaxed mind. Through practice, the joints, internal organs, and glands are all strengthened. The Chi Gung approach to exercise is thus radically different from the typical Western approach. In my 30 years of experience in the martial arts and in Oriental healing I saw at least a thousand practitioners of Chi Gung who were as relaxed, flexible, and capable at the age of 80 as is the average 20- to 30-year-old.

The fundamental methodology of Chi Gung involves the use of the chi to activate the body's internal pumping mechanisms for the purpose of moving bodily fluids more efficiently. Chi Gung exercises are, in effect, the energetic equivalent of pumping iron.

The body, being mostly fluids, has several internal pumping mechanisms besides the cardiovascular system (the cerebrospinal system, for example). Chi Gung works by increasing the flow of chi to these internal pumps. Blood, which carries oxygen and nutrients to the body's cells and removes their waste products, is perhaps the most important body fluid. Chi Gung has methods for moving blood through the veins and arteries just as strongly as does Western-style aerobics, but without strain. Rather than solely emphasizing cardiovascular-pulmonary exercises, Chi Gung contains specialized motions for the liver, kidneys, spleen, and various glands and nerves.

Chi Gung may be practiced standing still, moving, sitting, or lying down. Of the many Chi Gung systems in China, the one probably most familiar to the West is Tai Chi Chuan, but many of the exercises in this book (such as the Eight Pieces of Brocade, the Five Animal Play, and the *Yijinjing*) are equally well known in China, where Chi Gung is now enjoying a revival, with 60 to 70 million followers. Most Chinese who practice do so to be vibrantly healthy or to cure specific diseases; many who practice are older people who are experiencing the realities of aging and want to do something about it. While in some regions Chi Gung is taking on the character of a revivalist religious movement (with healing through the laying on of hands), simultaneously whole clinics, hospitals, and exercise centers are being devoted to advancing the health benefits of Chi Gung from a scientific point of view.

The computer revolution has become possible because ways have been found to pass electricity between all parts of the computer hardware with greater and greater efficiency. The Chinese have long recognized that, by increasing and balancing the power of the chi in the body, a similar positive revolution can occur within the individual. Currently, Chi Gung represents a new frontier in Western medicine. As time passes, and the concepts and principles of Chi Gung become understood in Western terms, this ancient way of keeping fit will bring health benefits throughout the Western Hemisphere. That, at least, is my fervent hope.

– Kumar Frantzis
Fairfax, California

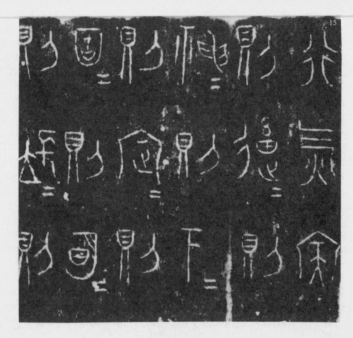

Illustration 1

A section of "On Breathing Exercise" inscribed on a piece of jade during the Warring States Period (475–221 B.C.). The whole text reads: "This calls for a round of deep breathing. Draw a deep breath and conduct it downward for storage, extension, fixation and consolidation. Then the air will grow up like a sprout and circulate in your body until it reaches the top of your head. Thus, you are identifying yourself with heavenly essence up above and earthly essence down below. One who goes along with this law of Nature would live, and one who goes against it would die."

Preface

This album contains 30 sets of physical exercises practiced by ancient Chinese, all taken from classical works or relics. Most of them are illustrated from the original sources, and we have reproduced the clear pictures and re-drawn the unclear ones. For those exercises with only instructions but no illustrations, new pictures have been drawn with the performer dressed in ancient costume.

The present is born out of the past. The health-preserving regimens we are using today are a development of those used by our ancestors, and a better understanding of the latter will help improve the former. A collection of illustrated ancient exercises will be of use to those who practice and study modern therapeutical exercises.

It was with this in view that some time ago Hai Feng Publishing Co. Ltd. entertained the idea of publishing such a book and asked us to compile it. We accepted the assignment with pleasure, but not without misgivings. We had seen a few ancient illustrations, but it would be no easy task to compile a whole book with the raw materials scattered in an ocean of archives covering thousands of years. Besides, we had little time to make an intensive study of the abstruse terms in the classic works. The collection would inevitably be far from complete and our interpretations could hardly be free from errors. We are saying all this in hope that our readers would not take it for an idle pretext.

Zong Wu & Li Mao
Beijing, 1991

Introduction

Mankind has known how to keep fit since the primeval days. Yet in different civilized societies fitness exercises may vary appreciably against different geographical and ideological backgrounds. More than four thousand years ago, according to historical records, the Middle Kingdom—as China has always been called—was hit by frequent torrential rains and floods. People suffered a lot from unbroken spells of wet weather. In order to relax their stiffened bones and muscles and dispel their gloomy moods, they would dance a kind of dance that could "conduct" (*daoyin*) the flow of blood and air (*qi**) in the body. Down through the ages, almost all the physical exercises were associated with *daoyin* and *qi*. The rubbing (Illustration 1) shows the inscription on a piece of jade during the Warring States period (475 – 221 B.C.) telling us how to conduct the air we breathe in, while Illustration 2 (page 210) shows a painting on silk unearthed from a tomb of the Western Han Dynasty (206 B.C. – A.D. 24), in which some people are doing *daoyin* exercises.

Later on, *qi* became a philosophical term with a much broader sense than the air we breathe in. According to ancient Chinese philosophy, it refers to the primordial for all living things in the universe. The *qi* in the human body is identified with the *qi* in the external world and falls into two categories, the prenatal *qi* and the postnatal *qi*. The former is the motive force of human life, consisting of *jingqi* (essential energy), which takes shape during the formation of the fetus, and *yuanqi* (primordial energy), which is cultivated in the process of pregnancy. The postnatal *qi* is the source of nourishment of human life, consisting of *tianqi* (heavenly *qi*), which goes to the lungs, and *diqi* (earthly *qi*), which goes to the stomach. The prenatal *qi* and postnatal *qi* act on each other to form *zhenqi* (genuine *qi*) for the vital activities. All physical exercises are based on this theory of integration of the universe and man and aim to cultivate and consolidate the genuine *qi* in the human body.

In ancient times, people held that the heaven had three essentials, namely, the sun, the moon and stars; the earth had three essentials, namely, water, fire and wind; and the human body also had three essentials, namely, *jing* (essence), *qi* and *shen* (spirit or mentality). As distinguished from modern Western physical exercises, the traditional Chinese physical exercises mobilize not only the bones, muscles and

---

* qi = chi

ligaments externally, but also the aforementioned three essentials internally, among which mentality plays the dominant role. For only when the mind is concentrated and attains perfect tranquility will *qi* be conducted into the "lower elixir field"—located in the lower belly and also known as "ocean of *qi*"—and flow freely to other parts of the body through a network of channels called *jingluo*. Then there are the analogous terms of *yin* and *yang* that frequently appear in this book. In the Chinese language, *yin* originally meant the shady side and *yang* the sunny side of anything under the sun. They were used by ancient Chinese thinkers for the two opposites that exist in all matters in the universe, for example, *yin* for the earth and *yang* for the heaven, *yin* for the feminine and *yang* for the masculine, *yin* for the negative and *yang* for the positive. The ancient physicians also held that there are *yin* and *yang* elements in the human body, which must be kept in balance. In the final analysis, all fitness exercises are aimed at the maintenance of this balance as a prerequisite for normal physiological functions and resistance to ailments.

Under the influence of various centuries-old schools of thought, particularly of Taoism, the ancient Chinese regimens have developed into present-day *qigong* exercises, which are gaining great popularity in China and abroad. But all the modern forms are still based on the traditional concept of unity between universe and man and between body and mind. The basic features of the ancient exercises, as can be observed in the 30 typical sets contained in this book, are still there, namely, a combination of mobility with immobility, of external with internal work, of bodily movements with respiration (and sometimes with self-massage), of health-preserving and longevity with prevention and treatment of diseases, and of the physical and moral aspects of keeping fit.

Most of the ancient exercises are simple and easy to learn. You may choose one or two sets for regular practice, taking into account your fitness level. As long as you persist and do the exercises properly, they will help you in improving health, curing disorders and living a long life. Their real value has already been proved in the past and will never be reduced with the passage of time.

(1) Chi Songzi's Physical and Breathing Exercises

This set of exercises is taken from *Dao Zang*, a collection of Taoist scriptures compiled during the period from the Six Dynasties (220 – 589) to the first half of the eighth century, and supplemented during the Song (960 – 1279) and Ming (1368 – 1644) dynasties.

This routine is named after Chi Songzi, a mythical figure who taught God of Farming the supernatural power of keeping alive in fire. Another source says he was a mortal being named Huang Chuping, who lived in the Jin Dynasty (265 – 420). Once while tending sheep, he was brought by a Taoist into a stone cabin on Mount Jinhua, where he became a fairy* by feeding on pine resin and a medical herb called "fuling" (*Poris cocos*) in reddish brown. Hence his alias Chi Songzi, meaning "red pine nut." He evolved a set of physical and breathing exercises for long life and good health. Fairy or no fairy, Chi's work has existed for at least 16 centuries.

Form 1

Kneel on a cushion with knees shoulder-width apart, soles facing upward, hands hanging at sides, head kept erect, eyes looking ahead and *qi* concentrated in lower elixir field.[†] Raise hands slowly to chest level, arms stretched and palms facing downward, and then to shoulder level, where they pause for a second or two, palms facing forward and fingers pointing outward. Move hands sideways in a downward arc before they are brought up to front of chest. Seven reps.[‡]

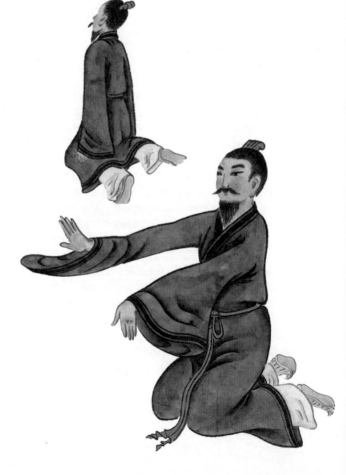

* fairy = immortal
[†] the area located in the upper ⅔ of the line joining the umbilicus and symphysis pubis.
[‡] reps = repetitions
Note: See Glossary, pp. 210 – 211, for definitions of unfamiliar terms.

Form 2

Take kneeling position as described above. Place hands on hips, thumbs pointing forward or backward, or with arms against sides and palms facing outward. Keep shoulders dropped and arms relaxed, with *qi* concentrated in lower elixir field and mind perfectly calm. Inhale through nose and exhale through mouth in six deep breaths.

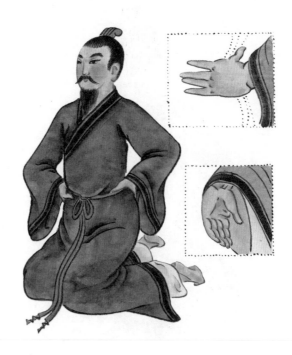

Form 3

Take kneeling position as described above. Place right hand on hip and move left arm, fully stretched, as high as possible behind back, where it pauses for 3 – 5 seconds before it is placed on hip while right arm is moved behind. Seven reps.

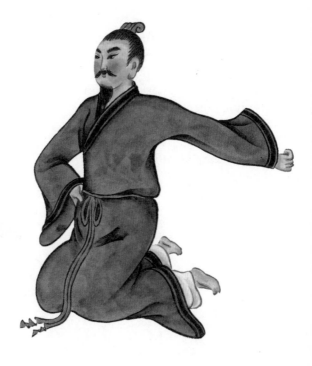

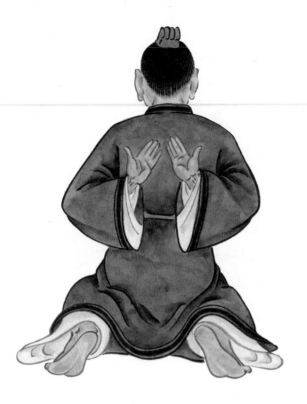

Form 4

Take kneeling position as shown. Bring both hands slowly behind and place them on back, palms facing outward and as near nape as possible, where they pause for 3 – 5 seconds before they are brought down to starting position. Seven reps, inhaling through nose when raising hands and exhaling through mouth when bringing them down.

Form 5

Sit on a cushion with legs stretched in front wider than shoulders; knees and toes turned outward, hands placed on hips, thumbs pointing forward and elbows turned a bit to front. Keep head erect, eyes looking ahead. Inhale through nose and exhale through mouth in deep, even, fine breaths.

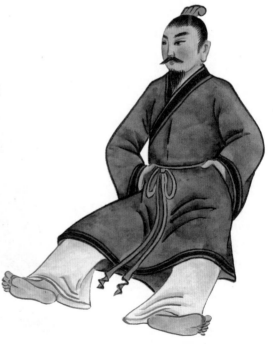

(2) Ling Jianzi's Physical and Breathing Exercises in Six Forms

This set of *daoyin* exercises in sitting position was created by Xu Xun (239 – 374), who was also known by his Taoist name of Ling Jianzi, meaning "Sacred Sword," and who, as legend has it, flew to heaven with his family on the last day of his mundane existence. The set was later collected into *Eight Essays on Health Preserving* by Gao Lian in the Ming Dynasty (1368 – 1644).

Form 1

Breathe out hot air into palms and rub cheeks up and down 30 – 50 times. Do this after meals and your face will never wrinkle but shine with health. This massage also cures eye diseases.

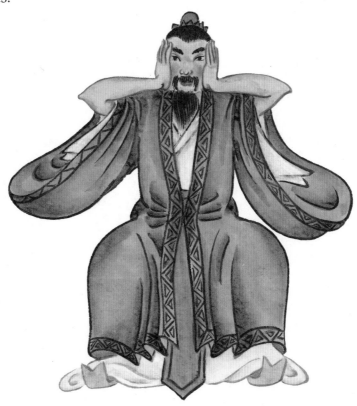

Form 2

Hold back of head with both hands and turn head round and round to facilitate circulation of blood in cranium and rid chest and back of pathogenic wind.* With fingers interlocked at nape, sway trunk ten times from side to side to rid bone joints of pathogenic wind. This exercise helps cure pulmonary disorders.

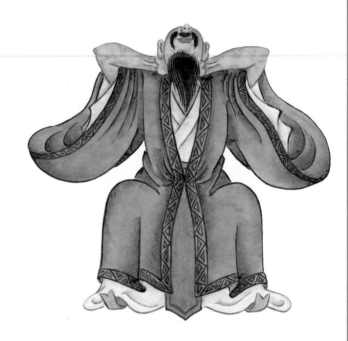

Form 3

Throw back head held by one hand and push one knee held by other hand. Do this with hands and legs alternated. 15 reps. This will clear blood vessels and rid bone joints of pathogenic wind that causes kidney and bladder troubles.

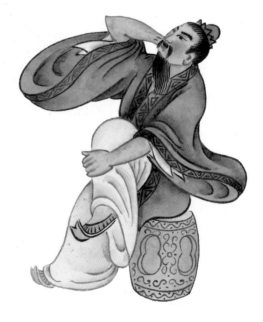

* There are five pathogenic factors according to traditional Chinese medicine, namely, wind, cold, dampness, mist and improper diet.

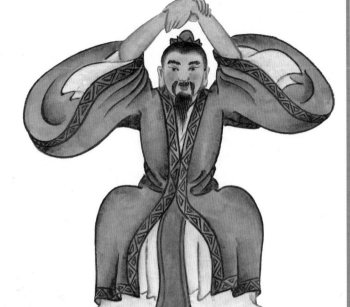

Form 4

With one hand holding the other wrist, extend arms overhead 15 times to get rid of spleen diseases.

Form 5

With one foot on floor and sole of other foot held in hands, try to extend raised leg 35 times. Do the same with feet alternated. This exercise will relieve lumbar strains, remove cold from kidneys and allay pains in knees.

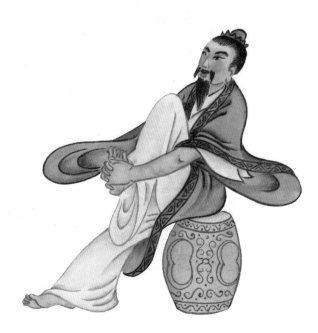

Form 6

Do the same as in Form 5 except that raised foot is held in hands by toes. Regular practice will rid kidneys of pathogens and cure emotional stress, beriberi and footsore after a long walk.

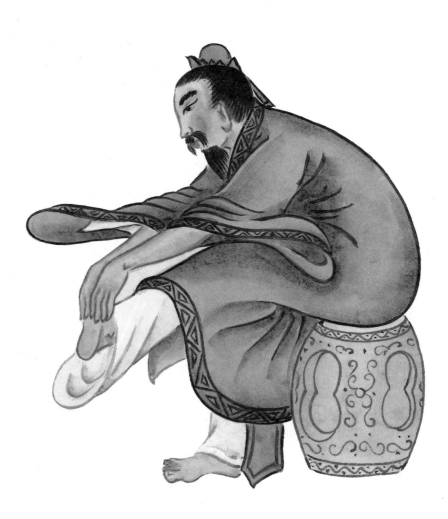

(3) Peng Zu's Physical and Breathing Exercises

This set of exercises is taken from *Yun Ji Qi Qian*, a collection of Taoist scriptures in seven parts compiled by Zhang Junfang during the Song Dynasty (960 – 1279). It is named after Peng Zu, who was born during the Xia Dynasty (21st – 16th century B.C.) and, as legend has it, lived to a ripe old age of 800 years, well into the Shang Dynasty (16th – 11th century B.C.).

The exercises are to be done from midnight to cockcrow, after a self-massage all over the body and on an empty stomach.

Form 1

Loosen garment and lie on back, legs stretched and feet shoulder-width apart, arms at sides, and eyes closed. Take five deep breaths.

This exercise is intended to activate *qi* in kidneys for a good balance between *yin* and *yang*.

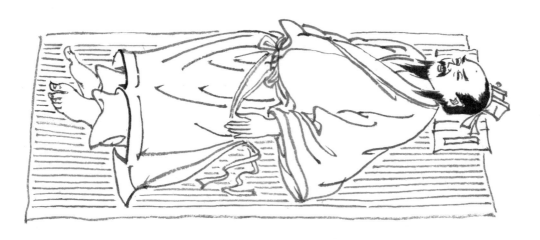

Form 2

Lie on back and hold toes as you take five deep breaths.

This exercise is intended to activate *qi* in the abdomen for the benefit of the "nine orifices," namely, two eyes, two ears, two nostrils, the mouth, the anus and the urethra (including the vagina).

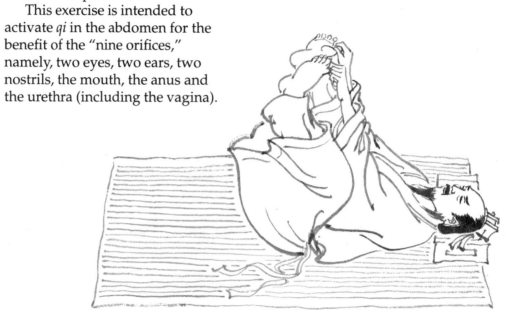

Form 3

Lie on back, arms placed on lower belly. Bend toes forcibly again and again as you take five deep breaths.

To improve the functions of kidneys and ears.

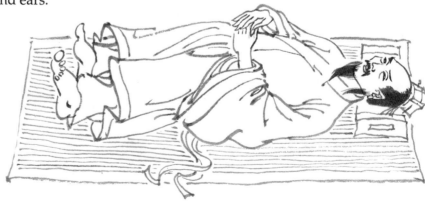

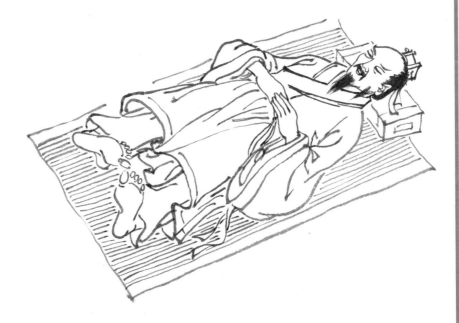

Form 4

Lie on back, left palm overlying right palm on lower elixir field, feet shoulder-width apart and toes turned inward. Take five deep breaths.

To cure coughing with dyspnea due to adverse ascending of *qi* in the lungs.

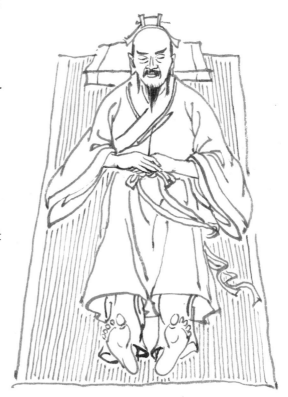

Form 5

Same as Form 4 except that feet are turned outward.

To rid the intestines and stomach of pathogenic factors (see footnote on p. 8).

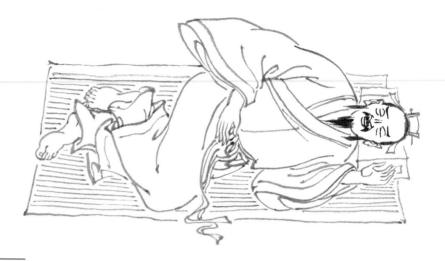

Form 6

Lie on left side, right foot placed behind left calf. Take five deep breaths.

To make up for deficiency of *qi* due to pathogenic wind and to improve eyesight.

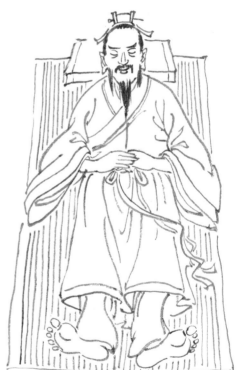

Form 7

Same as Form 4 except that toes are turned outward with feet in dorsal position.

To make leg muscles and ligaments flexible.

Form 8

Lie on back and hold knees in
front of chest as you take five deep
breaths.
   As a cure for backache.

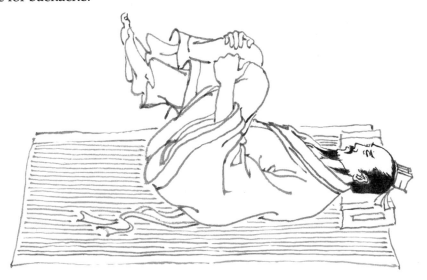

Form 9

Lie on back and rotate feet ten
times.
   For muscle strains.

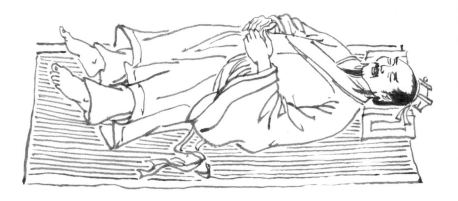

Form 10

Sit upright facing east, hands on knees. After holding breath for a while, raise arms and sway trunk from side to side, like willow branches swaying in a gentle breeze. Do this as long as you think fit.

To improve eyesight, keep hair black and cure disorders caused by pathogenic wind in the head.

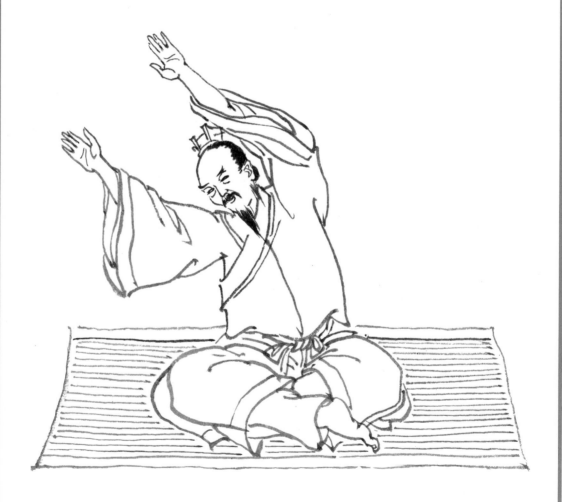

(4) Monk Xuanjian's Physical and Breathing Exercises

Also taken from *Yun Ji Qi Qian.*

Form 1

Sit with legs crossed, hands holding nape of neck. Bend forward — until forehead touches ground, if possible — as you take five deep breaths.

As a cure for shortness of breath.

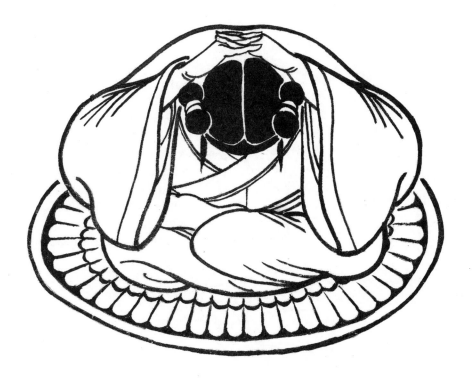

Form 2

Sit with legs crossed, left palm on lower elixir field and right palm on left palm. Take five deep breaths through nose. Do this with palms alternated.

For pathogens in large intestines.

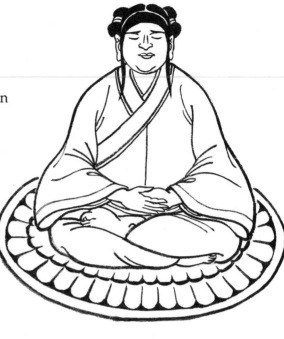

Form 3

Sit with legs crossed. Raise left hand, fingers pointing up, while right palm is placed on ground. Take five deep breaths through nose. Do this with hands alternated. Eyes follow raised hand.

For hypochondriac lumps.

Form 4

Sit with legs crossed, left hand akimbo* and right hand raised, fingers pointing up, as you take five deep breaths. Do this with hands alternated.

For pathogens in small intestines.

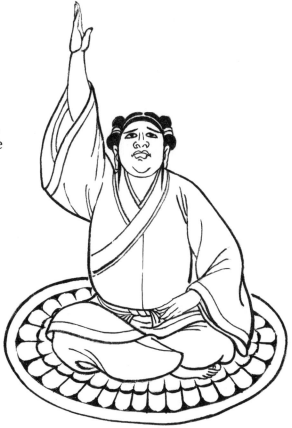

19

Form 5

Sit with legs crossed, head lowered, palms placed on left knee, as you take five deep breaths. Circle head clockwise over knees five times. Do this with palms placed on right knee.

For strains in lumbar vertebrae.

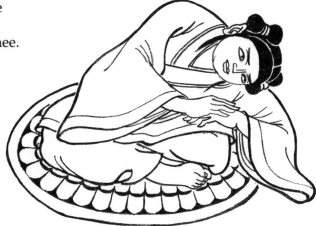

*akimbo = hand on hip, elbow out

Form 6

Sit with legs crossed and both hands on left part of chest, fingers interlocked. Move hands in five clockwise circles, right elbow raised. Starting from right part of chest, move hands in five counter-clockwise circles.

For pathogens in shoulders.

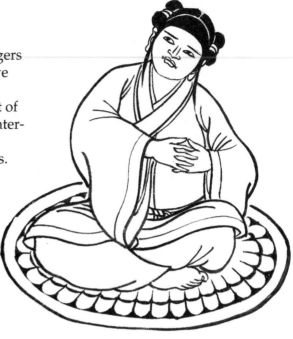

Form 7

Sit with legs crossed, hands holding nape of neck. Sway trunk from side to side as you take five deep breaths.

For pathogens in head.

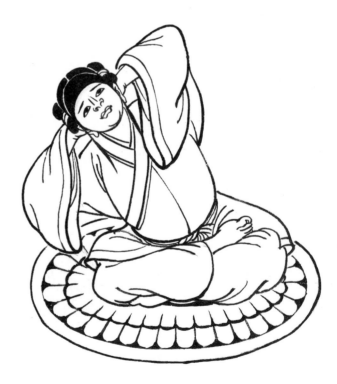

Form 8

Sit with legs crossed and hands
akimbo. Bend trunk to right and
left as you take five deep breaths.
      For discomfort in chest.

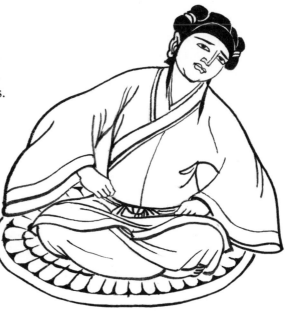

Form 9

Sit with legs crossed and fingers
interlocked. Move hands to left
and right and lower head over
knees as you take five deep
breaths.
      For strains in shoulders.

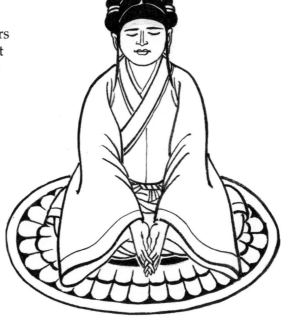

Form 10

Sit with legs crossed. Raise both hands overhead five times, each with a strug of shoulders.
　For itching skin.

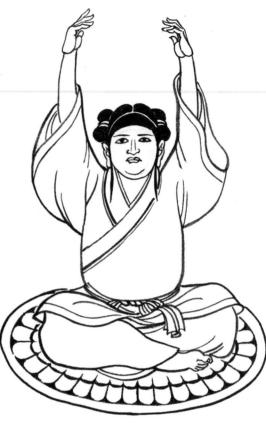

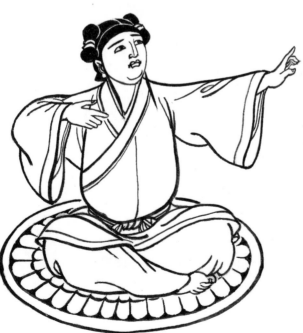

Form 11

Sit with legs crossed. Raise left arm sideways and bend right arm at elbow as if in act of drawing the bow. Do this with arms alternated. Five reps.
　For stagnation of *qi* in shoulder blades.

Form 12

Stand with one foot in front
of the other, palms on lower
belly. Stamp feet alternatively,
with greater force for front
foot, moving trunk to and fro.
Change position of feet. 27
reps.

For stagnation of *qi* and
cold in spleen, and many
other diseases.

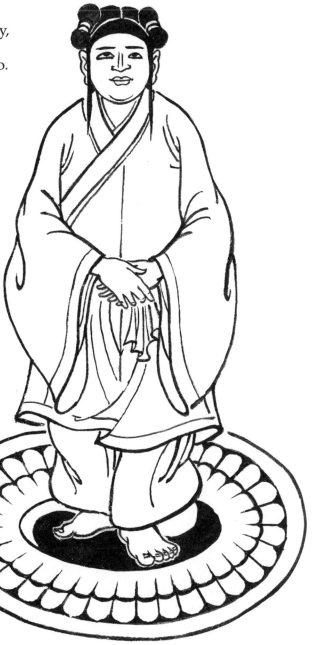

(5) Chen Xiyi's Physical and Breathing Exercises in Sitting Position

Chen Xiyi, a Taoist in the 10th – 11th century, worked out this set of *daoyin* (physical and breathing) exercises to be done at different hours in different periods of the year. In the traditional Chinese calendar, the solar year is divided into 24 periods, with a solar term for the first day, while the day is divided into 12 periods, each covering two hours and called an earthly branch.

Chen's work was later collected into two books published in the Ming Dynasty (1368 – 1644), namely, *Health Preserving* and *San Cai Tu Hui (Drawings of the Heaven, Earth and Man)*.

Form 1
For First Half of First Moon

This period begins with the Day of Beginning of Spring, which falls on February 3, 4 or 5 of the solar calendar. The exercise is to be done at a time covering the first two earthly branches, that is, between 11 o'clock at night and 3 o'clock in the morning.

Sit with legs crossed in front and palms on right thigh, one overlying the other. Turn trunk and head to right with a shrug of right shoulder and then to left with a shrug of left shoulder. 15 reps. Cool-down exercise: Strike upper and lower teeth three times, take three breaths "to get out the stale and take in the fresh," and gargle throat with saliva three times.

As a cure for disorders caused by retention of pathogenic wind (see footnote on p. 8) in abdomen, retroauricular pains, and aching back, shoulder, arm and elbow.

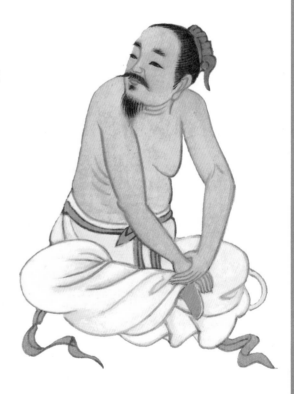

Form 2
For Second Half of First Moon

This period begins with the Day of Rain Water, which falls on February 18, 19 or 20. The exercise is to be done at 1 – 3 o'clock in the morning.

Sit with legs crossed in front and palms placed on right thigh, one overlying the other. Turn trunk and head to right and left without shrugging shoulders. 30 reps. Cool-down exercise as in Form 1.

For disorders caused by pathogenic factors (see footnote on p. 8) in the triple warmers,* dry sensation in pharynx, hiccup due to cold in stomach, inflammation of throat, deafness, excessive sweating, outer canthus and pain in cheeks.

*The upper, middle and lower warmers housing some of the internal organs and also functioning as passageways of *qi* and fluids.

25

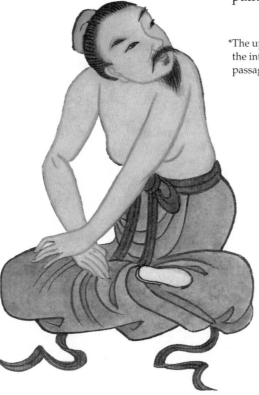

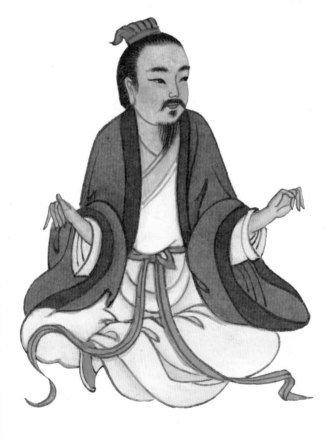

Form 3
For First Half
of Second Moon

This period begins with the Day of Waking of Insects, which falls on March 5, 6 or 7. The exercise is to be done at a time covering the second and third earthly branches, that is, between 1 – 5 o'clock in the morning.

Sit with legs crossed in front and arms bent at sides, hands half clenched. Turn head to right and left as you push both elbows backward. 30 reps. Cool-down exercise: Strike upper and lower teeth 36 times, take nine breaths "to get out the stale and take in the fresh," and gargle throat with saliva nine times.

For disorders caused by pathogenic factors in lumbus, paravertebral musculature of back, lungs and stomach; jaundice, dry mouth, nose bleeding, inflammation of throat, swollen face, sudden loss of voice, gingival atrophy, photophobia, and loss of smelling senses.

Form 4
For Second Half
of Second Moon

This period begins with the Day of Spring Equinox, which falls on March 20 or 21. The exercise is to be done at 1 – 5 o'clock in the morning.

Sit with legs crossed in front. Thrust arms forward as you turn head to right and left. 42 reps. Cool-down exercise as in Form 3.

For disorders caused by pathogenic factors in *jingluo* channels in chest, shoulders and back; toothache, swollen neck, shivering with cold, deafness, itching, tinnitus, retroauricular pain, and aching back, shoulder, arm and elbow.

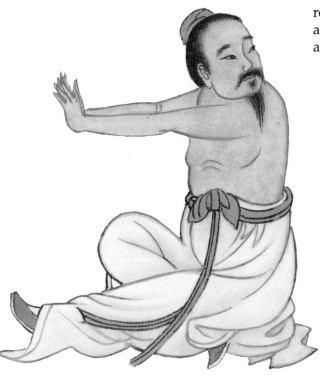

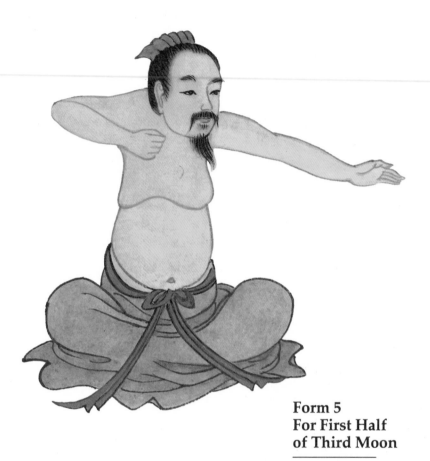

Form 5
For First Half
of Third Moon

This period begins with the Day
of Pure Brightness, which falls on
April 4, 5 or 6. The exercise is to
be done at 1 – 5 o'clock in the
morning.

Sit with legs crossed in front.
Draw an imaginary bow with
right hand. Change hands.
42 reps. Cool-down exercise as
in Form 1.

For disorders caused by
pathogenic factors in lumbus, kidneys, intestines and stomach,
preauricular heat, pharyngalgia,
pains in neck, shoulder, arm and
elbow, and debility of limbs.

Form 6
For Second Half
of Third Moon

This period begins with the Day of Grain Rain, which falls on April 19, 20 or 21. The exercise is to be done at 1 – 5 o'clock in the morning.

Sit with legs crossed in front. Raise right hand overhead, arm stretched and palm up, while left arm is bent across chest. Change hands. 35 reps. Cool-down exercise as in Form 1.

For blood stasis in spleen and stomach, jaundiced eyes, nose bleeding, swollen cheeks and jaws, pains in arms, elbows, buttocks, and excessive heat in palms.

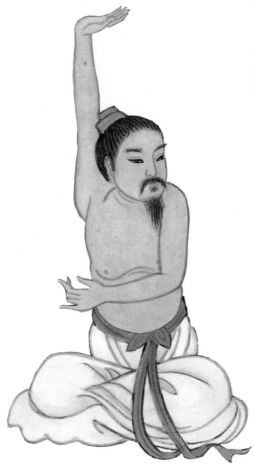

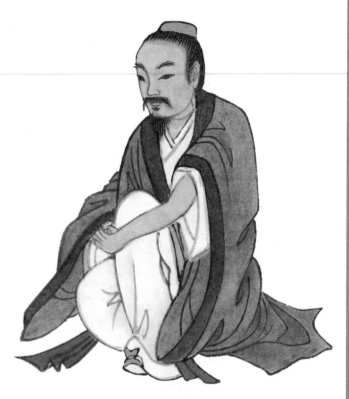

Form 7
For First Half
of Fourth Moon

This period begins with the Day of Beginning of Summer, which falls on May 5, 6 or 7. The exercise is to be done at a time covering the third and fifth earthly branches, that is, at 3 – 7 o'clock in the morning.

Sit with legs crossed in front and eyes closed. Raise left knee and hold it back forcibly with both hands, holding breath for a moment. Do the same with right knee. 35 reps. Cool-down exercise as in Form 1.

For disorders caused by pathogenic wind and dampness, pains in *jingluo* channels, contracture or subjective sensation of contraction in arm and elbow, swelling of axilla, excessive heat in palm, and susceptibility to excessive joy.

Form 8
For Second Half
of Fourth Moon

This period begins with the Day of Grain Full, which falls on May 20, 21 or 22. The exercise is to be done at 3 – 7 o'clock in the morning.

Sit with legs crossed in front. Raise right hand overhead, arm stretched and palm up, while left hand presses downward. Change hands. 15 reps. Cool-down exercise as in Form 1.

For disorders caused by pathogenic factors in internal organs, fullness in chest and hypochondrium, severe palpitation, flushed face, jaundiced eyes, irritability, precordial pain, and excessive heat in palms.

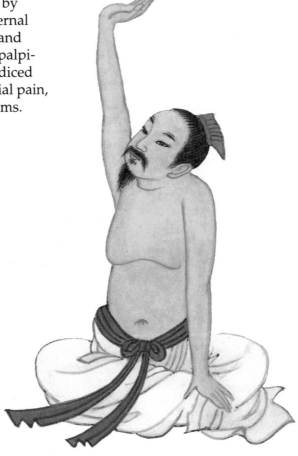

Form 9
For First Half
of Fifth Moon

This period begins with the Day
of Grain in Ear, which falls on
June 5, 6 or 7. The exercise is to be
done at 3 – 7 o'clock in the
morning.

Stand with trunk leaning back
and both hands raised, palms up.
Raise one hand further up while
bringing other hand down to
front of shoulder. Change hands.
35 reps. Cool-down exercise as in
Form 1.

For consumptive diseases of
lumbus and kidneys, dry
sensation in pharynx, precordial
pain, dipsesis, jaundiced eyes,
flushed face, pain in hypochondrium, diabetes, susceptibility to excessive joy and fright,
coughing, vomiting, diarrhea due
to stagnation of *qi*, pain in thigh
due to fever, precordial pain,
headache, pain in neck, and
flushed face.

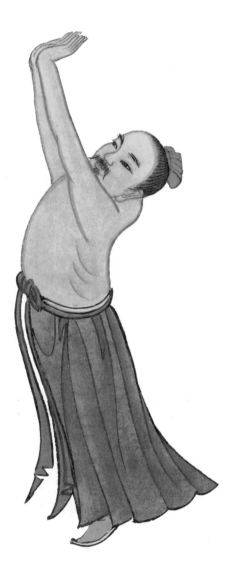

Form 10
For Second Half
of Fifth Moon

This period begins with the Day
of Summer Solstice, which falls on
June 21 or 22. The exercise is to be
done at 3 – 7 o'clock in the
morning.

Sit with legs bent in front.
Hold right foot with hands, and
push it forward forcibly. Change
feet. 35 reps. Cool-down exercise
as in Form 1.

For disorders caused by
pathogenic wind and dampness,
pains in wrist, knee, arm, back
and kidney, excessive heat in
palms, and sensation of heaviness
in limbs.

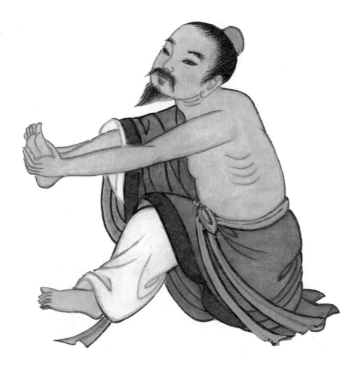

Form 11
For First Half
of Sixth Moon

This period begins with the Day of Slight Heat, which falls on July 6, 7 or 8. The exercise is to be done at 1 – 5 o'clock in the morning.

Kneel with trunk leaning back and hands supporting on floor. Stretch right leg. Change legs. 15 reps. Cool-down exercise as in Form 1.

For disorders caused by pathogenic wind and dampness in leg, knee and lumbus, distension and fullness in lungs, dry sensation in pharynx, asthma, pain and swelling in supra-clavicular fossa, pain in abdomen, spasm of hand, sensation of heaviness in limbs, hemiplegia, hemiapoplexy, amnesia, asthma, proctoptosis, debility of wrists, and susceptibility to changing moods.

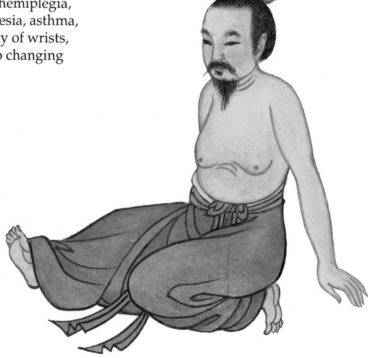

Form 12
For Second Half
of Sixth Moon

This period begins with the Day of Great Heat, which falls on July 22, 23 or 24. The exercise is to be done at 1 – 5 o'clock in the morning.

Sit with legs crossed in front and both hands holding legs. Turn head to right and left, like a tiger eyeing its prey. 15 reps. Cool-down exercise as in Form 1.

For disorders caused by pathogenic wind in head, neck, chest and back, coughing, abnormal rising of *qi*, asthma, irritability, fullness in chest and hypochondrium, excessive heat in palms, pains in shoulder, upper arm and back, sweating due to pathogenic wind and cold, apoplexy, oliguria, loose stool, dermic pain and numbness, susceptibility to sorrow, and feeling of cold or heat all over body.

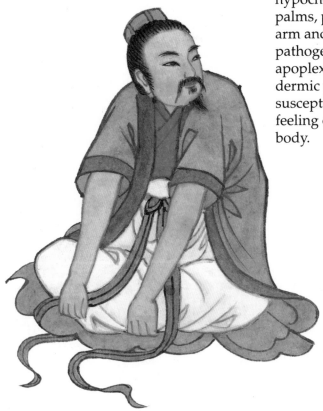

Form 13
For First Half
of Seventh Moon

This period begins with the Day of Beginning of Autumn, which falls on August 7, 8 or 9. The exercise is to be done at 1 – 5 o'clock in the morning.

Kneel with hands supporting on floor. 56 shrugs of shoulders. Cool-down exercise as in Form 1.

For disorders caused by *qi* deficiency and pathogenic factors in lumbus and kidneys, bitter taste caused by disorders of liver and gallbladder, susceptibility to melancholy, pains in heart and hypochondrium making lying on side difficult, dusty complexion, headache, pain in jaws, outer canthus, swelling in supraclavicular fossa and armpit, and sweating while shivering with cold.

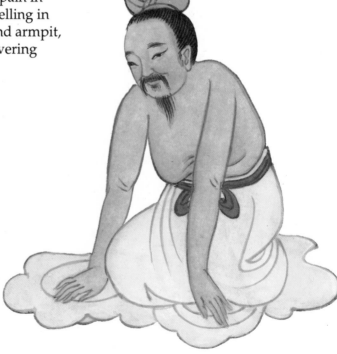

Form 14
For Second Half
of Seventh Moon

This period begins with the Day of Limit of Heat, which falls on August 22, 23 or 24. The exercise is to be done at 1 – 5 o'clock in the morning.

Sit with legs crossed in front. Turn head to right and left as you tap back with both hands. 35 reps. Cool-down exercise as in Form 1.

For disorders caused by pathogenic wind and dampness, pains in shoulder, back, chest, calf and ankle, and coughing and asthma.

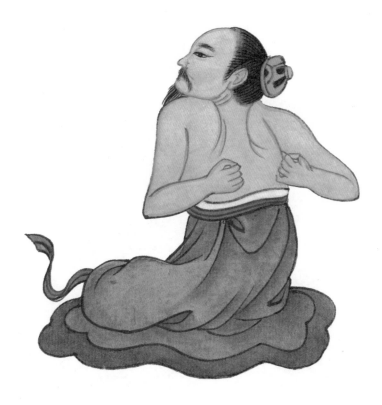

Form 15
For First Half
of Eighth Moon

This period begins with the Day of White Dew, which falls on September 7, 8 or 9. The exercise is to be done at 1 – 5 o'clock in the morning.

Sit with legs crossed in front, hands on knees. Turn head to right and left. 15 reps. Cool-down exercise as in Form 1.

For disorders caused by pathogenic wind and dampness in *jingluo* channels in back, sweating while shivering with cold, nosebleeding, facial hemi-paralysis, dry sore on lips, swollen neck, inflammation of throat, sudden loss of voice, dark complexion, vomiting, frequent yawning, dementia causing wild singing and desire to run nude.

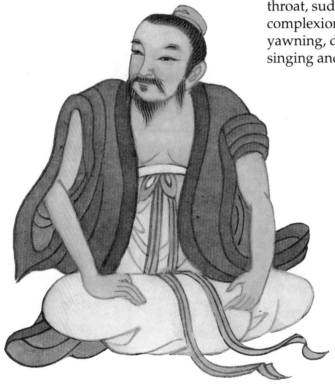

Form 16
For Second Half
of Eighth Moon

This period begins with the Day of Autumnal Equinox, which falls on September 22, 23, or 24. The exercise is to be done at 1– 5 o'clock in the morning.

Sit with legs crossed in front, hands covering ears and elbows pointing sideward. Bend trunk to right and left. 15 reps. Cool-down exercise as in Form 1.

For disorders caused by pathogenic wind and dampness, edema in chest, back and abdomen, swelling and pains in leg, knee, ankle and instep, stiffness of thigh, strain in upper arm, enuresis due to *qi* deficiency, polyorexia, asthma, and cold in stomach.

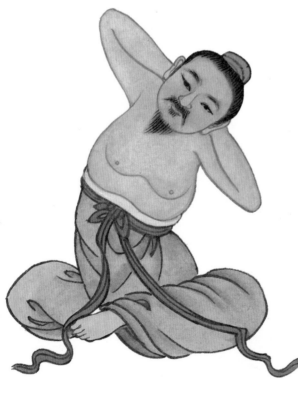

39

Form 17
For First Half
of Ninth Moon

This period begins with the Day of Cold Dew, which falls on October 8 or 9. The exercise is to be done at 1 – 5 o'clock in the morning.

Sit with legs crossed and both hands raised, palms up. Raise both hands 15 times. Cool-down exercise as in Form 1.

For disorders caused by pathogenic wind, cold and dampness in *jingluo* channels of hypochondrium, headache, outer canthus, neck and back pain, piles, dementia, jaundiced eyes, nosebleeding, and cholera.

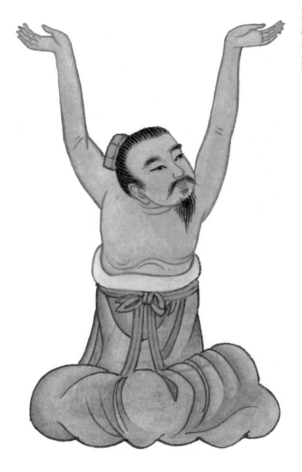

Form 18
For Second Half
of Ninth Moon

This period begins with the Day of Frost's Descent, which falls on October 23 or 24. The exercise is to be done at 1 – 5 o'clock in the morning.

Sit with legs bent in front, holding feet with hands separately. Push feet with force. 35 leg pushes. Cool-down exercise as in Form 1.

For disorders caused by pathogenic wind and dampness in lumbus and foot, stiffness of thighbone and knee joint, strain in upper arm, pains in neck, back, hip and leg, flaccidity of muscles, passing stool with blood and pus, ardor urine, distension and pain in abdomen, cold feet, and prolonged piles and proctoptosis.

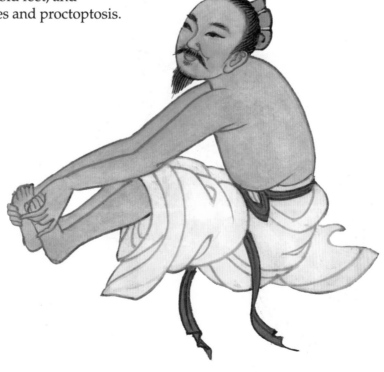

Form 19
For First Half
of Tenth Moon

This period begins with the Day of Beginning of Winter, which falls on November 7 or 8. The exercise is to be done at 1 – 5 o'clock in the morning.

Sit with legs crossed in front. Push hands to right and left as head turns to opposite side. 15 reps. Cool-down exercise as in Form 1.

For disorders caused by pathogenic factors and consumptive diseases in chest, backache making trunk bend difficult, dry sensation in pharynx, dusty and pallid complexion, sensation of fullness in chest and limbs, vomiting, poor appetite, headache, dizziness, eye sore, deafness, swollen cheeks, and pain in abdomen.

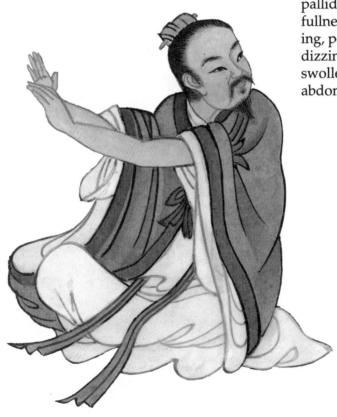

Form 20
For Second Half
of Tenth Moon

This period begins with the Day of Slight Snow, which falls on November 22 or 23. The exercise is to be done at 1 – 5 o'clock in the morning.

Sit with legs crossed in front. Place left hand on left knee while right hand holds left elbow to pull it forcibly inward. Change hands. 15 reps. Cool-down exercise as in Form 1.

For disorders caused by pathogenic wind, dampness and heat in internal organs, swelling of lower belly for women, swelling and pain or nodulation and numbness of scrotum for men, pain in testicles or penis, inguinal hernia, dysuria, urinary disorders, and susceptibility to fright.

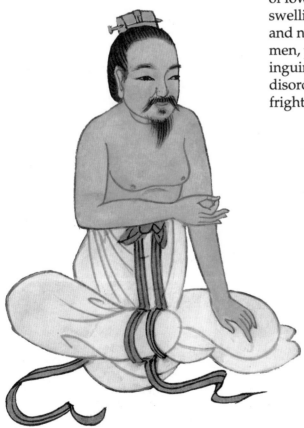

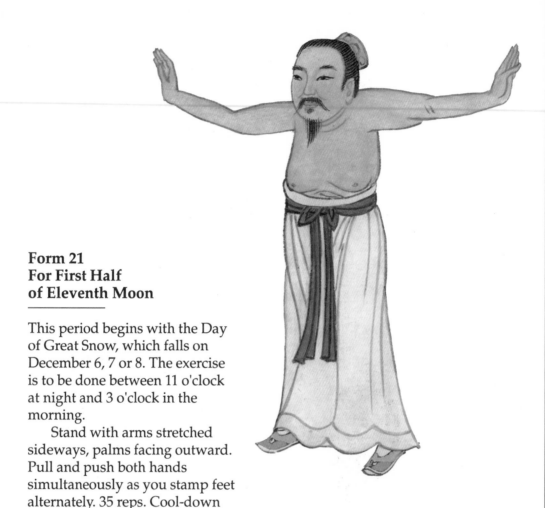

Form 21
For First Half
of Eleventh Moon

This period begins with the Day of Great Snow, which falls on December 6, 7 or 8. The exercise is to be done between 11 o'clock at night and 3 o'clock in the morning.

Stand with arms stretched sideways, palms facing outward. Pull and push both hands simultaneously as you stamp feet alternately. 35 reps. Cool-down exercise as in Form 1.

For disorders caused by pathogenic wind and dampness in knee and foot, dryness of tongue, inflammation of pharynx, abnormal rising of *qi*, irritability, precordial pain, jaundice, spouting bleeding from anus, frequent urination, poor appetite, dark complexion, hemoptysis, coughing with dyspnea, poor eyesight, and susceptibility to fright.

Form 22
For Second Half
of Eleventh Moon

This period begins with the Day of Winter Solstice, which falls on December 21, 22 or 23. The exercise is to be done between 11 o'clock at night and 3 o'clock in the morning.

Sit with legs stretched in front. Press knees forcibly with separate hands. 15 times. Cooldown exercise as in Form 1.

For disorders caused by pathogenic cold and dampness in *jingluo* channels of four limbs, pains in back, hip, shoulder, thigh and abdomen, sleepiness, sensation of fullness in chest, constipation, dysentery, chilblain, cold and swelling in lower back, and reversed flow of *qi* under navel.

45

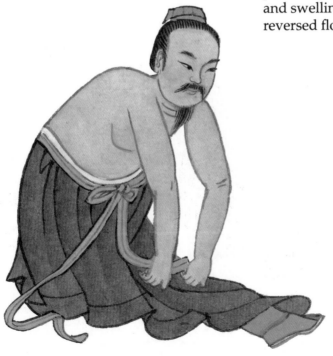

Form 23
For First Half
of Twelfth Moon

This period begins with the Day of Slight Cold, which falls on January 5, 6 or 7. The exercise is to be done between 11 o'clock at night and 3 o'clock in the morning.

Sit with legs crossed in front. Press left knee with left hand while raising right hand overhead, arm stretched and palm facing upward. Change hands. 15 reps. Cool-down exercise as in Form 1.

For nausea, pain in stomach, distension in abdomen, poor appetite, diarrhea, sensation of heaviness in limbs, precordial pain, irritability, jaundice, constipation, oliguria, frequent thirst, lassitude and sleepiness.

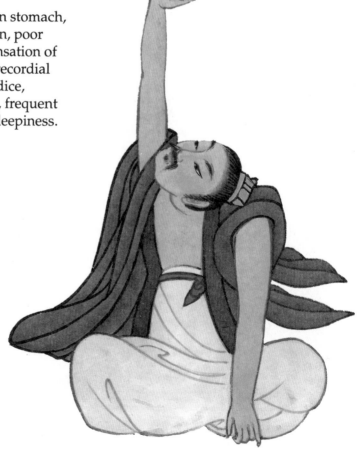

Form 24
For Second Half
of Twelfth Moon

This period begins with the Day of Great Cold, which falls on January 20 or 21. The exercise is to be done between 11 o'clock at night and 3 o'clock in the morning.

Kneel with hands on floor supporting trunk from behind. Stretch legs alternately with as much tension as feels comfortable. 15 reps. Cool-down exercise as in Form 1.

For disorders caused by stagnation of *qi* in *jingluo* channels, pain at root of tongue, debility of body, swollen hips and knees after standing for a while, pains in back, buttocks, upper arm, calf and foot, distension in abdomen, borborygmus, indigestion, edema of foot, and obstruction in the "nine orifices," namely, two eyes, two ears, two nostrils, the mouth, the anus and the urethra (including the vagina).

(6) Wang Ziqiao's Physical and Breathing Exercises

Wang Ziqiao, as legend has it, was a princess in the sixth century B.C. who spent three decades meditating in the Songshan Mountains and flew into Heaven as a fairy. This set of exercises was collected into *Dao Zang*, an encyclopedia of Taoism.

The whole set contains 34 forms, of which 20 are selected here.

Form 1

Sit on a mat with legs stretched in front, feet shoulder-width apart. Move arms behind, palms on mat and thumbs spread out and pointing sideward. Shift weight of trunk gradually onto arms and close eyes lightly. Inhale slowly through mouth and exhale through nose.

As a cure for disorders in chest.

Form 2

Sit upright with legs crossed and hands akimbo, thumbs pointing backward and shoulders dropped. Lower head slowly as you exhale through mouth (above) and throw head back slowly as you inhale through nose (below). 30 reps.

For dizziness.

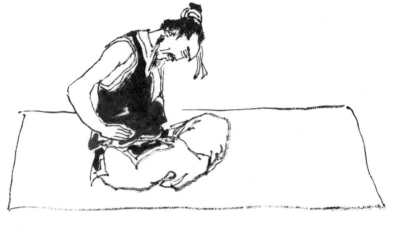

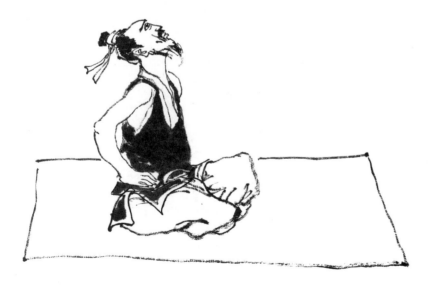

49

Form 3

Sit upright with legs crossed, left palm on lower elixir field and right hand pinching nose. Inhale through nose as you release right hand and exhale through mouth. Do this until you begin sweating lightly.

For dim eyesight, dacryorrhea and headache due to cold.

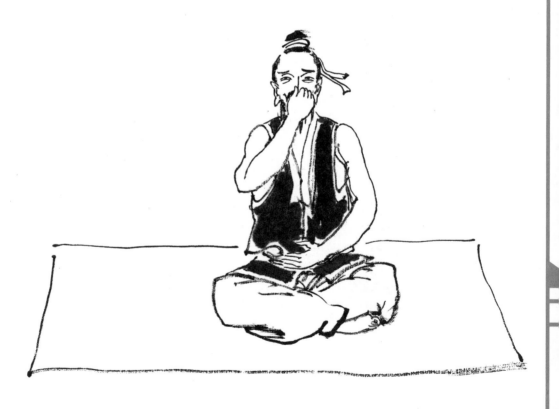

Form 4

Sit upright with legs crossed.
Move hands to front of belly,
palms up and corresponding
fingers pointing at each other.
Raise them to chest level and,
with an internal rotation of
arms, further up overhead,
palms up and corresponding
fingers pointing at each other.
Eyes follow hands. Inhale
deeply through nose when
you raise hands; hold breath
for a moment while hands
stay overhead. Move hands
slowly back to starting
position as you exhale through
mouth. Seven reps.

For abdominal masses.

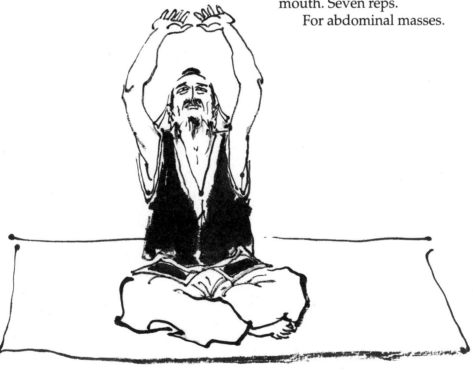

Form 5

Sit upright with legs crossed.
Raise left hand overhead past
belly and chest, palm up and
fingers pointing backward, while
right palm rests at side on mat.
Pause for a while and do the same
with hands alternated. Seven reps.
Inhale through nose when raising
hand and exhale slowly through
mouth when lowering it.

For pains in arms and abdominal disorders due to stagnation
of *qi*.

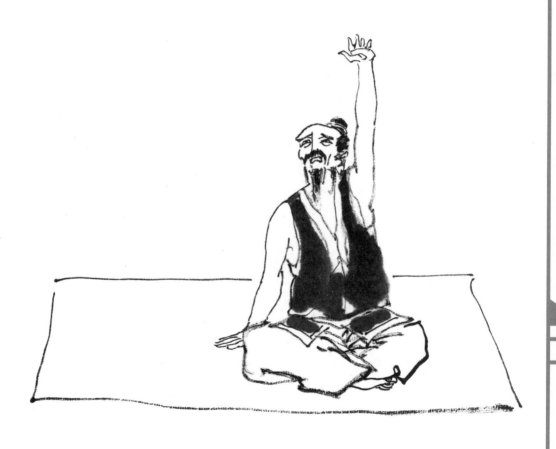

Form 6

Sit upright with knees raised and legs crossed, hands joined around shins and fingers interlocked. Inhale through nose and hold breath as your abdomen heaves up and down 14 or 21 times before you exhale through mouth. Seven reps.

This exercise promotes circulation of blood and *qi* and persistent practice makes old people look younger.

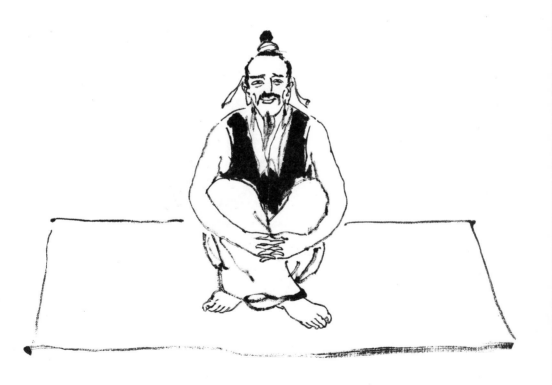

Form 7

Sit upright with legs crossed and left palm pressed against lower belly, right palm on left palm. Bend trunk slowly to left and right as you take seven breaths, inhaling through nose and exhaling through mouth.

For disorders caused by attack of pathogenic wind (see footnote on p. 8) on the head.

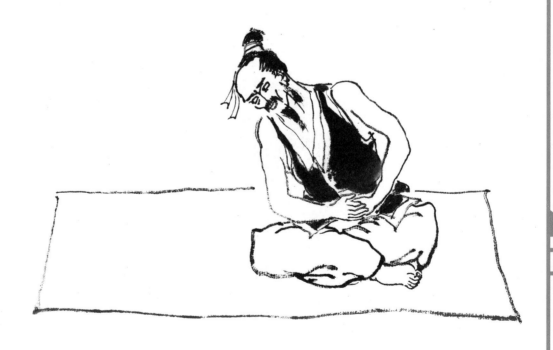

Form 8

Sit upright with legs crossed and hands akimbo, thumbs pointing forward, as you take dozens of breaths, inhaling through nose and exhaling through mouth.

For abdominal distension due to overeating as well as abdominal disorders caused by pathogenic cold.

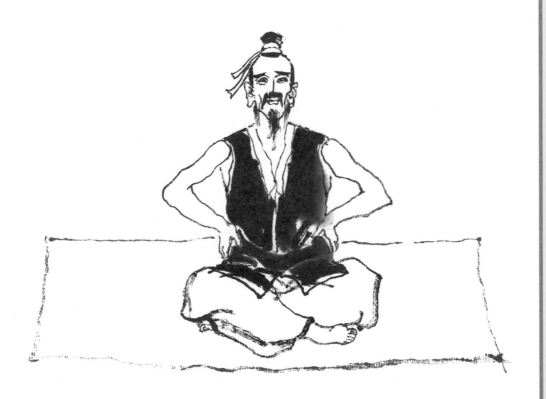

Form 9

Sit upright with legs crossed. Turn head to right as you stretch right arm fully sideways at shoulder level, forefinger pointing up and thumb spread out, while left hand is placed in front of left shoulder, palm inward and elbow thrust forcibly sideways. Do this with arms alternated. Seven reps. Inhale through nose when raising arms and exhale through mouth when lowering them slowly.

For uncomfortable feelings in four limbs, irritability and backache.

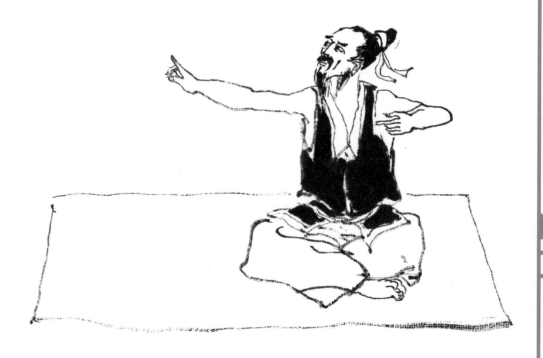

Form 10

Sit with legs crossed. Raise right
hand overhead, palm up and
fingers pointing backward, while
left palm is placed under right
armpit. Put down hands at waist
sides. Seven reps. Inhale through
nose when raising hands, and
exhale through mouth when
putting them down.

For pathogenic cold in
stomach and abdominal
disorders.

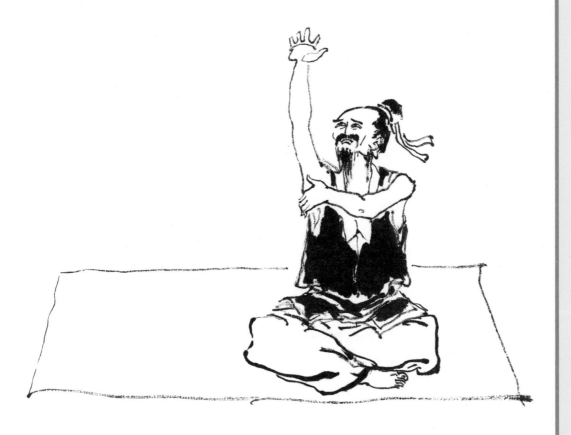

Form 11

Repeat movements in Form 10 with hands alternated.

    For blood stasis and stagnation of *qi*.

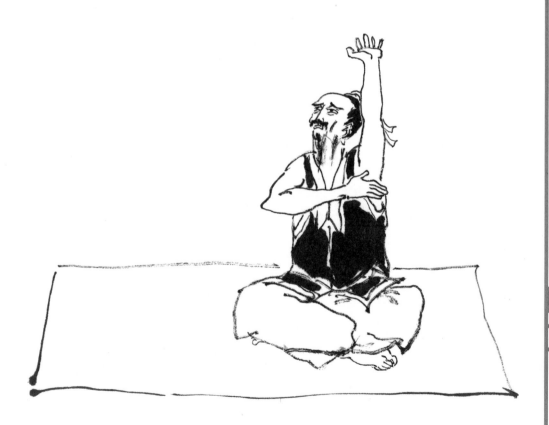

Form 12

Sit with legs crossed. Place palms
behind, arms bent, shoulders
relaxed, head thrown back and
eyes half closed. Hold this
position as you take dozens of
breaths.

   To rid pathogenic heat and
repair dead tissues.

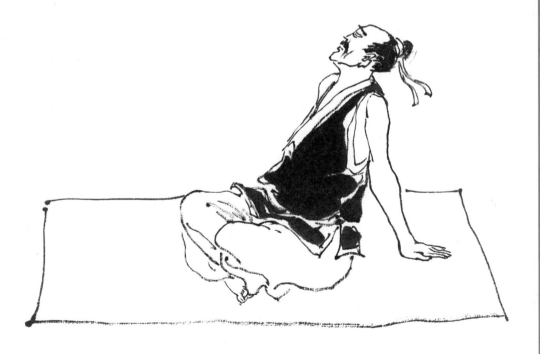

Form 13

Sit in kneeling position,* with
knees raised a bit and held in
separate hands as you take seven
deep breaths, inhaling through
nose.

    For aching waist and back.

*Be very careful of your knees in this position,
especially if you have had knee problems. If
you feel any pain, ease back on the tension.

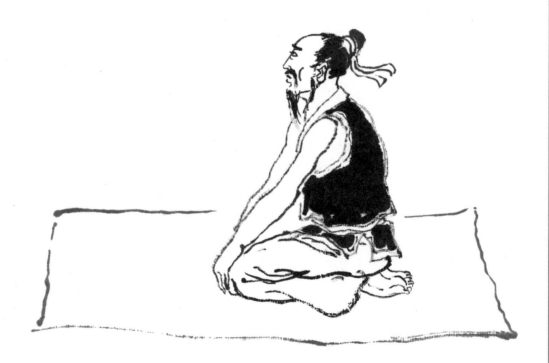

Form 14

Sit in kneeling position.* Hold
heels with separate hands as you
take seven deep breaths, inhaling
through nose.
    For vomiting.

*See note at left.

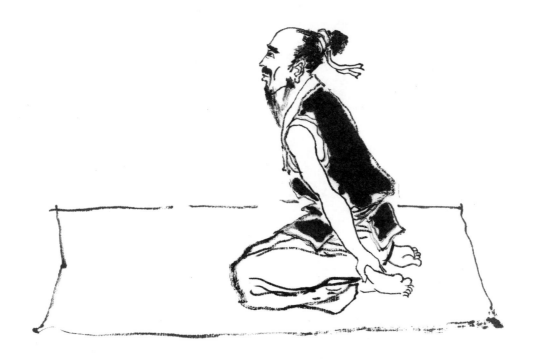

Form 15

Sit upright with legs crossed,
palms on knees. With focus of
attention on left part of body, turn
head to look to left. Hold this
position as you take dozens of
deep breaths.

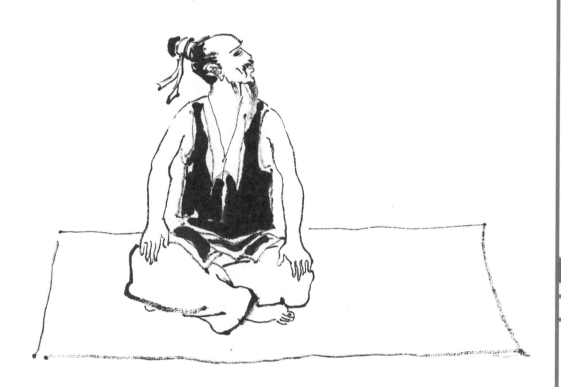

Form 16

Sit upright with legs crossed, palms on knees. With focus of attention on right part of body, turn head to look to right. Hold this position as you take dozens of deep breaths.

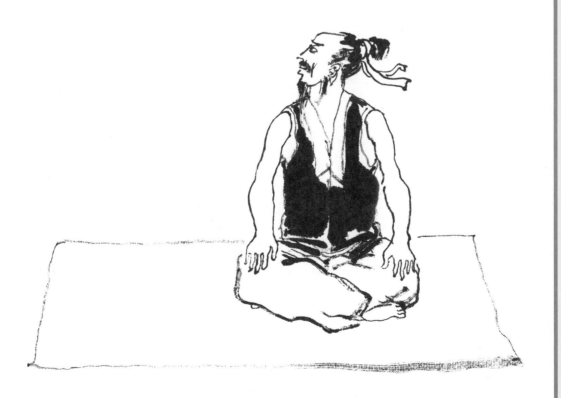

Form 17

Sit upright with legs crossed and palms on knees. If you feel a mass in abdomen, raise head toward the sun. Hold this position as you take dozens of deep breaths.

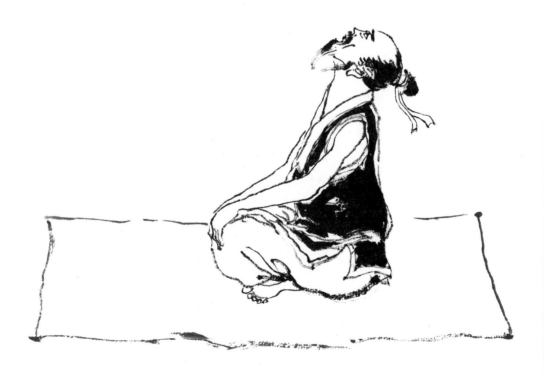

Form 18

Sit upright with legs crossed. Stretch right leg, toes turned outward, and raise left knee and hold it with both hands. Hold this position as you take seven deep breaths. Do same for other side.

For stiffness of four limbs and headache when getting up from bed.

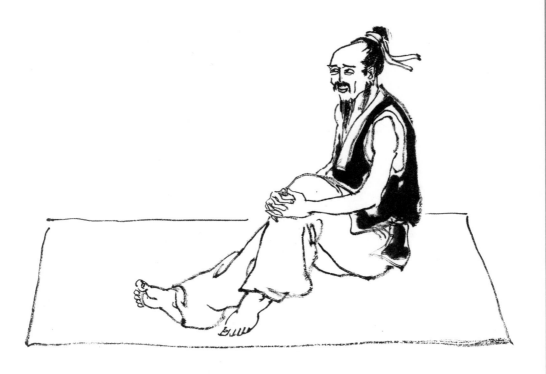

Form 19

Do the same as in Form 18, with
other leg.
    Also for dim eyesight and
deafness.

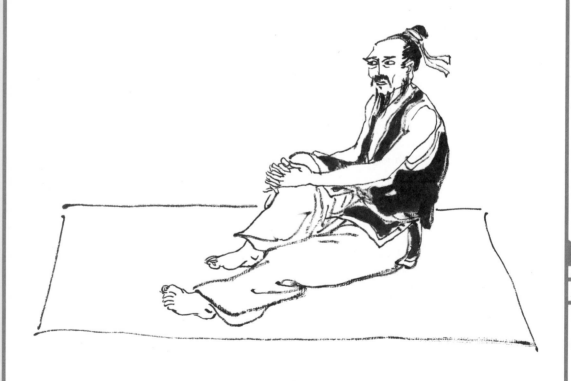

Form 20

Sit upright with legs crossed, eyes looking ahead. Bend trunk to left side, head supported on left palm, elbow on mat, while right arm lies on right side of body. Hold this position as you take dozens of breaths, inhaling slowly through mouth and exhaling slowly through nose. Do same on right side.

For depression and melancholy.

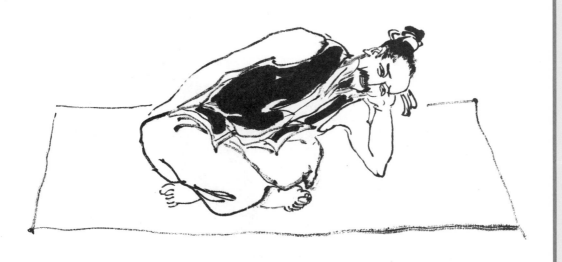

(7) The Five-Animal Play

The Five-Animal Play, initiated by Hua Tuo, a physician during the Eastern Han Dynasty (25 – 220), has developed into many styles down through the last 18 centuries. The one chosen here is taken from *Yun Ji Qi Qian*, a book published in the Song Dynasty (960 – 1279).

Form 1
Tiger's Play

Start with hands and feet on floor, head raised and eyes staring ahead. Take three steps forward, first with left hand and right foot and then with right hand and left foot; take three steps backward. Bend left arm and left leg for a side roll on floor to resume starting position. Do the same by reversing right and left. Repeat these movements until you begin sweating slightly. Breathe naturally throughout the exercise.

Imagine yourself as a powerful, fierce tiger descending a hill.

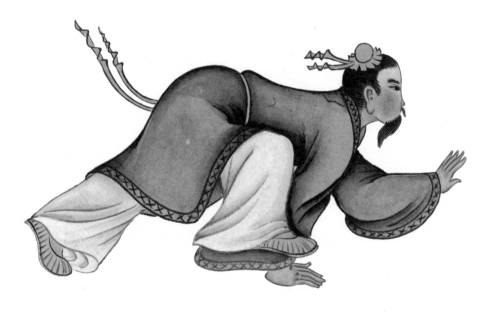

Form 2
Bear's Play

Lie on arched back, chins drawn
in and legs bent. Hold knees separately with hands and press them
backward, while raising trunk
and lowering head to shift body
weight onto buttocks; then lean
trunk backward and bring knees
close to chest, so as to rock
yourself to and fro, for as many
times as befits your physical
condition. Keep back arched all
the while to prevent head from
touching floor. Breathe naturally.

Imagine yourself as a bear
frolicking alone.

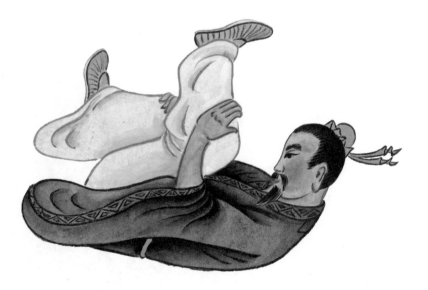

Form 3
Deer's Play

Bend trunk forward until hands
touch floor, neck craned. Turn
head to right to look back into distance, while stretching left leg
backward for a pause of two or
three seconds. Do the same by
reversing right and left. Repeat
these movements as many times
as befits your physical condition.
Coordinate them with respiration,
breathing in when turning head
backward, holding breath during
pauses and breathing out when
turning head to front.

Imagine yourself as a deer
standing at an elevated place,
sensing some imminent danger
and looking back into the
distance, only to find everything
clear.

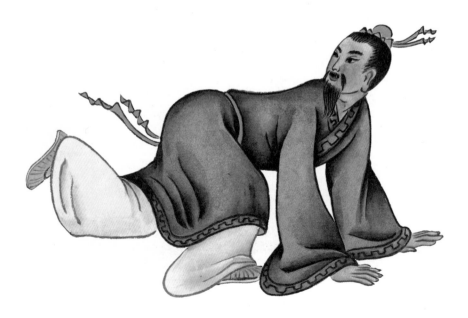

Form 4
Ape's Play

Stand with feet apart. Raise right hand overhead in form of a hook, arm slightly bent at elbow and fingers pointing downward, while left hand, also hooked, is placed in front of left part of chest, trunk stretched and right knee raised for a pause of two or three seconds. Put right foot down and bend both legs slightly, trunk shrunk with a forward lean; place both palms slowly in front of knees. Do this again by reversing right and left. Repeat these movements as many times as befits your physical condition Coordinate them with respiration, breathing in when stretching body, holding breath during pauses and breathing out when shrinking trunk.

Imagine yourself as an ape climbing up a tree branch and then climbing back down after gathering some fruit.

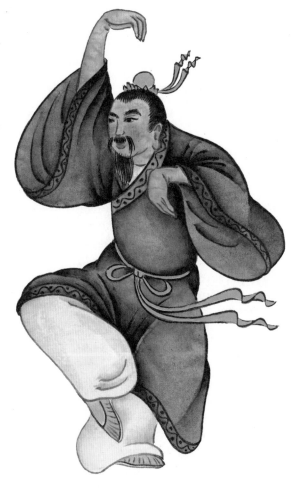

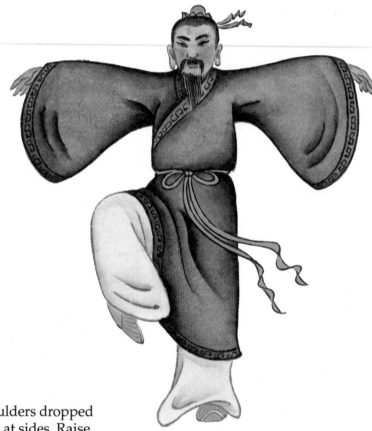

Form 5
Bird's Play

Stand at ease, shoulders dropped
and arms hanging at sides. Raise
arms sideways to shoulder level,
palms down, while right knee is
raised, left heel off floor. Put both
arms, left foot and right heel
down to resume starting position.
Do the same by reversing right
and left. Repeat these movements
36 times. Breathe in through nose
when raising arms and breathe
out through mouth when putting
arms and feet down.

    Imagine yourself as a bird
winging its way through the air.
Looking ahead gives you a
pleasant sense of traveling in
infinite space.

(8) A Rare Copy of the Five-Animal Play

This is a rare copy of the Five-Animal Play inscribed on a piece of brocade that has been handed down since the 10th century as an heirloom in Shen Shou's family in Zhejiang Province. It bears the words "A Genuine Heritage from Hua Tuo."

Form 1
The Pouncing Tiger

Imagine yourself as a fierce tiger in a tawny coat with black stripes, roaming in wilderness and ready to pounce on its prey.

(1) Starting position (for all forms): Stand upright with feet shoulder-width apart, toes pointing forward, arms hanging at sides, head kept erect, and eyes looking ahead.

(2) Turn right foot 45° outward with heel as pivot, and lift left foot to right ankle as you place hands beside ribs, in form of tiger's paws, palms down.

(3) Bend right leg at knee and take a stride forward to left with left foot; shift body weight onto left leg to form a left "bow step," with front leg bent and rear leg stretched. At the same time push both hands in a forward-upward-downward arc to stop in front of chest, arms slightly bent at elbow, just like a tiger ready to pounce on its prey. (See figure.)

(4) Repeat movements in step 3, reversing right and left.

(5) Do 1 – 3 series of the three forward steps. Then turn about on left to resume starting position and do the same number of series in reverse direction. There may be another round of the back-and-forth walking movements.

Essential points: Keep in mind the image of a pouncing tiger throughout performance, concentrating on its quality of powerfulness. When taking the bow step, movements should be unhurried but vigorous, with a calm but sharp look in eyes. Inhale in this phase of action and exhale when thrusting out paws, uttering a hushed sound of "ah" through half-opened mouth — a method of respiration often used in *qigong* exercises. The whole is actually an uninterrupted flow of tensions alternated with relaxation, a close coordination between external and internal movements of the body.

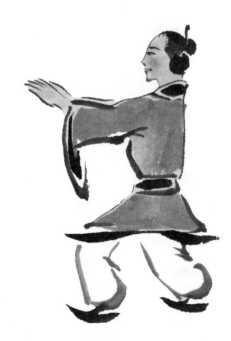

Form 2
The Running Deer

Imagine yourself as a deer roaming a grassland, turning its head now and then.

(1) Take a left bow step as does the Pouncing Tiger, but in a smaller stride and with a higher body position, toes turned only 30° outward. At the same time move left hand in a rightward-downward-forward arc to right front above head, fingers spread out and pointing up and palm facing inward — in imitation of a deer's horn; while right hand,

clenched loosely, swings in a rightward-backward-downward arc until back of fist touches coccyx, thumb side up — in imitation of a deer's tail.

(2) Turn trunk and neck to left — together with left arm — as far backward as possible, to cast a backward glance into distance. With horn remaining at same level, bend right wrist to raise tail. (See figure.)

(3) Repeat movements in 1 and 2, reversing right and left.

Essential points: The imaginary deer is supposed to be on the alert, with a watchful but kindly look in eyes. Yet the exercise should be performed in a quiet, self-contented mood, with light steps and relaxed joints, stressing softness in all movements. Hands should move in curved lines and body turn in a spiral. Inhale when raising arms and exhale when turning trunk, uttering a hushed sound of "hsu" through half-closed mouth. Movements of upper and lower limbs should be continuous and well coordinated.

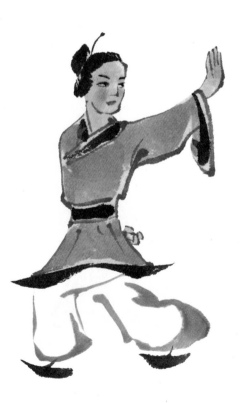

Form 3
The Frolicking Bear

Imagine yourself as a brown bear standing on hind legs on a rocky hill and playing under a pine tree, its forepaws clutching at low branches.

(1) Using waist as hinges, shake body rhythmically, with hands bent forcefully at wrist and legs slightly bent at knee.

(2) Shift weight onto right leg and take a forward step with left foot as does the Pouncing Tiger, but farther to left and with a half stride. At the same time move left hand in a horizontal circle counterclockwise — about 30 inches in circumference — at left side in front of body, no higher than navel.

(3) As above movements are going on one after another, bend right leg slightly at knee and withdraw right hand to waist side.

(4) Repeat movements in 2 and 3, reversing right and left and replacing counterclockwise with clockwise. (See figure.) Thus all the movements — with left or right hand, at higher or lower position, in clockwise or counter-clockwise circle, by bending or stretching limbs — conform to the philosophical principle of unity of two opposites, whether in terms of *yin* (negative) and *yang* (positive), or hardness and softness.

Essential points: All movements should hinge on waist. Arms should be bent with utmost force to mobilize muscle groups in shoulders, chest and back to the full. Inhale when moving left hand forward and exhale when moving right hand forward, utter-ing a hushed sound of "hu" through half-closed mouth.

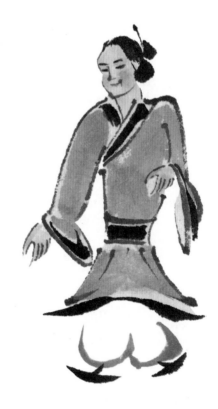

Form 4
The Romping Ape

Imagine yourself as a white ape perched on two branches, one higher than the other, gathering pears only to throw them away.

(1) Raise left knee to stand on right leg; at the same time raise left hand to right front, arm stretched and palm turned up, while right hand is brought down to back, fingers pointing down.

(2) Bend right leg for a squat and place left foot outside right foot to form a cross-step. At the same time turn left hand into fist as if to pick a fruit, and bring it to waist side with an internal rotation of arm; unclench fist and move arm down to back as if to throw something away. Meanwhile, move right hand up to right front and raise right knee to stand on left leg. (See figure.)

(3) Repeat movements in 2, reversing right and left.

(4) Eyes follow raising hand and give a few winks after gathering fruit.

Essential points: Every motion — a grab on the fruit, a cross-step in low profile, or a merry bat of the eyelids — should be nimble, with trunk kept erect all the while. Inhale when raising knee to stand on a single leg, and exhale when bending leg for a squat, uttering a hushed sound of "si" through clenched teeth.

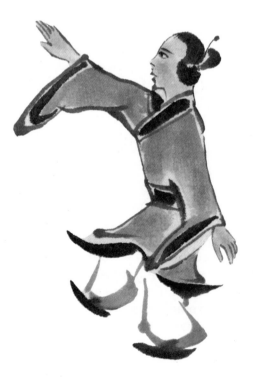

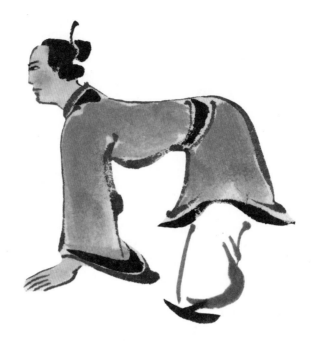

Form 5
The Swooping Bird

Imagine yourself as an owl swooping down on its prey on a moonlit night.

(1) Bend wrists to point fingers forward. Without turning body, move eyes in a clockwise circle to scan field ahead.

(2) Take a stride forward with left foot and follow it with right foot, as both hands move backward and then circle to front, arms stretched at shoulder level. Bend forward and support yourself with palms on floor and raise head to look ahead. (See figure.)

(3) Repeat movements in 1 and 2, replacing clockwise with counterclockwise and reversing right and left.

Essential points: The searching glance should be slow but cover a broad scope, lasting for a time taken by a single breath. Inhale when stepping forward and exhale when bending down, uttering a hushed sound of "chui" through flat lips, as you do when whistling.

(9) Zhou Lüjing's Five-Animal Play

This routine of Five-Animal Play is taken from *Yi Men Guang Du*, an encyclopedia compiled by Taoist Zhou Lüjing at the turn of the 17th century. The book is divided into 13 parts, including Classics, Common Knowledge, Hygiene, Food, Fauna and Flora. The five forms of exercises come from different sources.

Form 1
The Tiger

Stand at ease with feet shoulder-width apart. Bend trunk forward and place both hands in front of belly, assuming the awe-inspiring power of a tiger. Hold breath as you straighten body as if you were pulling up a heavy weight. Draw a deep breath into belly and breathe out slowly after a short pause. Five to seven reps.

This exercise is intended to activate your *jingluo* system, refresh your vigor and cure you of various illnesses.

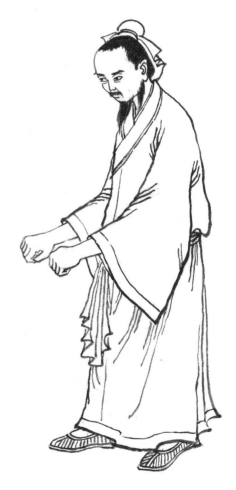

Form 2
The Bear

Stand at ease. Hold breath as you raise right fist overhead and place left fist in front of hip. At the same time swing up right leg sideways like a bear in wobbling gait. Sink air into right part of chest. After a short pause, place down right hand and foot as you exhale in a gentle breath. Do the same with left hand and foot. Three to five reps.

To relax your bones and ligaments, calm your mind and cultivate *qi* and blood.

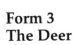

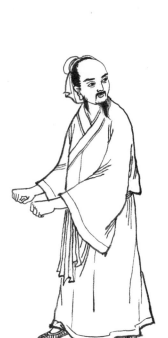

Form 3
The Deer

Stand at ease. Bend trunk a bit forward and place both fists in front of belly. Hold breath as you turn head back on left to look at buttocks like a deer casting a backward glance. At the same time raise both heels and put them down immediately to produce a shock through whole body; do this two or three times before taking another breath. Repeat these movements with head turned to opposite direction.

Form 4
The Ape

Stand at ease. Hold breath as you move right hand to front of belly as if to hold a branch, while left hand is raised as if to gather a fruit. At the same time raise both heels and turn head to right, as you sink air into belly. After a short pause, exhale in a gentle breath. Do the same by reversing right and left. Repeat these movements until you start sweating lightly.

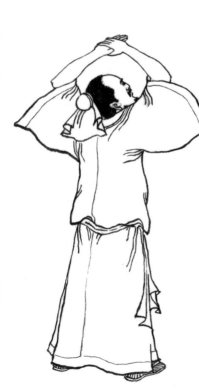

Form 5
The Bird

Stand at ease. Hold one hand with the other and raise them overhead, trunk kept erect and head thrown back, like a bird ready to take wing. Hold breath and visualize *qi* around coccyx rushing up to top of head. Pause for a while and do the same with hands alternated.

(10) Self-Massage

The following set of self-massage methods, taken from *Si Bu Cong Kan*, a four-part collection of classical works compiled by Zhang Yuanji (1867 – 1959), may have evolved before the 14th century. Practice it three times a day and you'll increase your appetite and improve your health in a single month.

Form 1

Wring and rub your hands as if you were washing them in a basin. This may be done in standing, sitting or lying position.

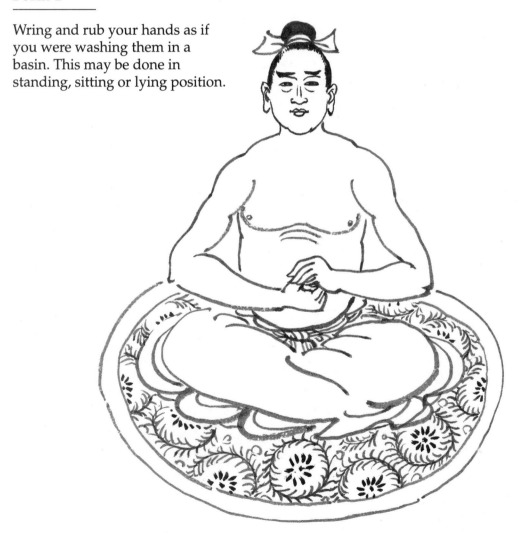

Form 2

Sit with legs crossed and fingers interlocked. Supinate and pronate* palms again and again.

*supinate = rotate hands so palms face forward
pronate = rotate hands so palms face chest

Form 3

Bend legs into semi-squat, fingers interlocked and placed on knees. Then with palms superimposed, circle knees as many times as you see fit, swaying trunk at the same time. Straighten body, raise left arm sideways to shoulder level while right arm is bent across chest, eyes looking to left side, as if in act of drawing the bow. Do this by reversing right and left. As many reps as you please.

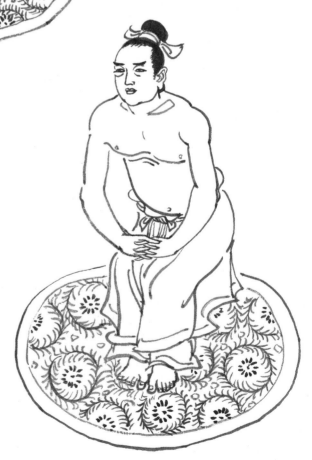

Form 4

Sit with legs crossed, hands clenched at sides, knuckles down. Thrust fists forward with an internal rotation of arms to turn knuckles upward. Withdraw fists to waist sides, knuckles down, and thrust them sideways, knuckles up. As many reps as you see fit.

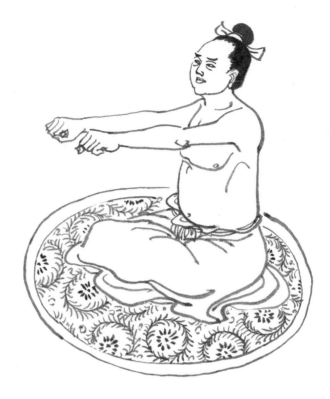

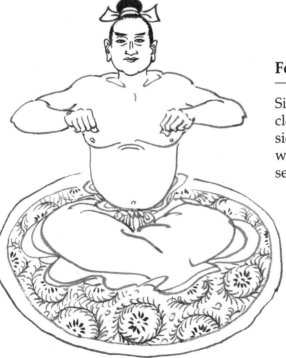

Form 5

Sit with legs crossed, hands clenched in front of chest, thumbs side up. Thrust elbows backward with a jerk. As many reps as you see fit.

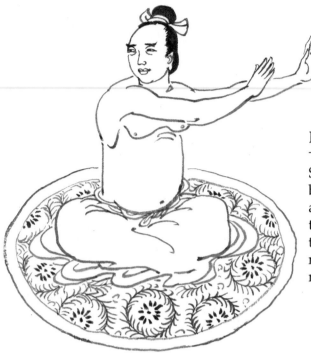

Form 6

Sit with legs crossed. Push
both arms forcefully to left
and right with a follow-
through of trunk, imagining
that you were pushing
mountains aside. As many
reps as you see fit.

Form 7

Sit with legs crossed, trunk
bent over knees and hands
holding back of head, fingers
interlocked. Shake trunk from
side to side several times.

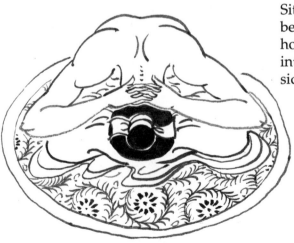

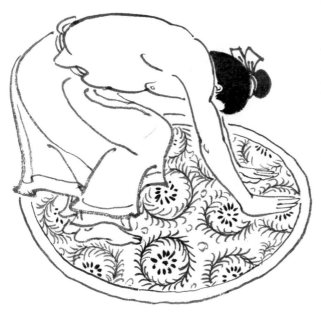

Form 8

With palms on ground and legs bent at knees, lift arched back three times. Tap spine with a stick or small club held in alternate hands, for any number of times.

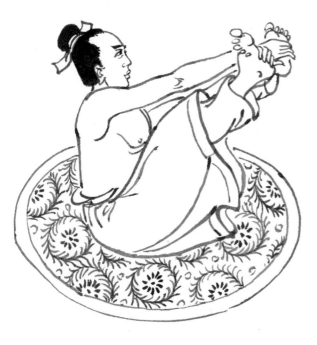

Form 9

Sit with legs raised and feet held in separate hands. Try to stretch legs three times, giving a stamping force against palms.

Form 10

With palms on ground
and legs bent at knee, lift
arched back three times as
you turn head to look
back.

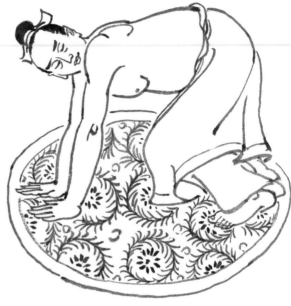

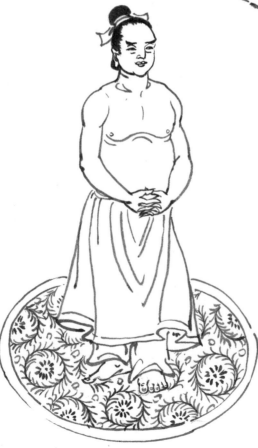

Form 11

Stand with hands on lower belly,
fingers interlocked and one foot
placed behind the other. Shift
body weight forward and
backward several times, with
heels of front and rear feet on and
off floor by turns. Do this with
feet in reversed position.

(11) Pu Qianguan's Massage for Longevity

Pu Qianguan, a pharmacologist and pathologist in the Song Dynasty (960 – 1279), advocated the good habit of doing physical exercises every day — in any place and at any time, just with some jerks of the body and limbs — bearing in mind the theory that flowing water is fresh and stagnant water is filthy. He also advised people to go to bed late and get up early in spring and summer, go to bed early and get up early in autumn, and go to bed early and get up late in winter — but on all occasions no earlier than cockcrow and no later than sunrise.

Before going to bed, one may take a "dry bath," that is, self-massage on arms (Figs. 1 – 2), on chest and belly (Fig. 3), and on legs (Fig. 4) — by running palms up and down a dozen times or so. After this, one may lie down on side and, with tongue touching palate, produce some saliva and swallow it before going to sleep.

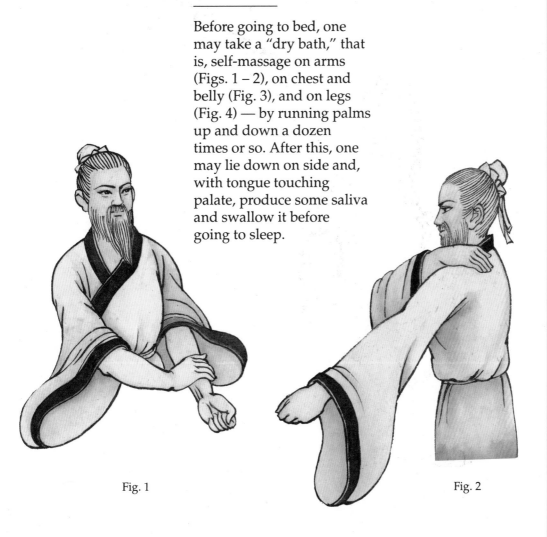

Fig. 1

Fig. 2

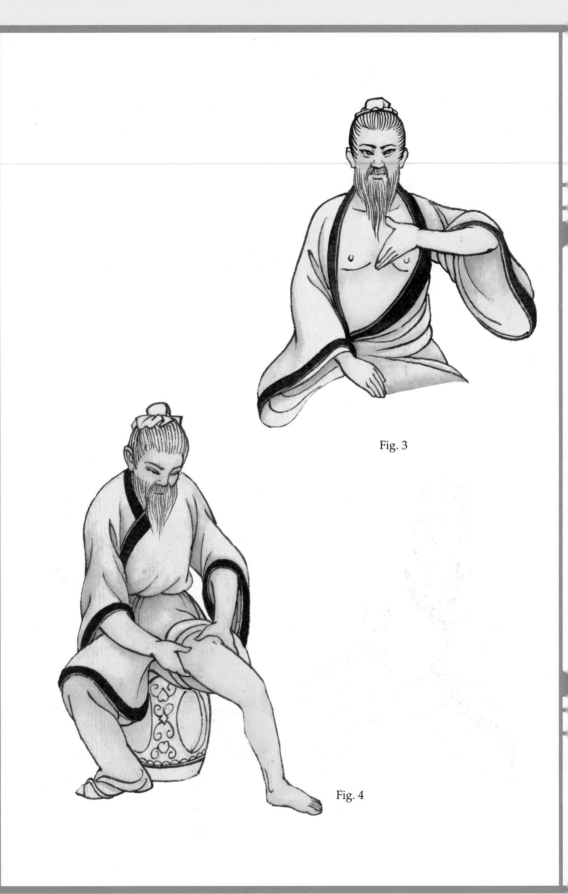

Fig. 3

Fig. 4

(12) Su Dongpo's Massage

This set of manipulations was created by Su Dongpo (1037 – 1101), well known not only as a man of letters, but also as a therapist. It is included in *Effective Recipes of Su and Shen*, a collection of prescriptions by Su Dongpo and his contemporary Shen Kuo (1039 – 1095) published in the Southern Song Dynasty (1127 – 1279). The exercises are to be done preferably in the wee hours of the morning.

Sit on a bed or stool, facing east or south. Strike lower teeth against upper teeth 36 times. Enter meditation with eyes closed and, with hands akimbo, take deep breaths through nose as you, with tongue pressed against teeth, produce plenty of saliva, which you swallow in three to five gulps. Rub hands warm and massage middle part of soles (Fig. 1), lower back on both sides (Fig. 2) and then face, eyes, ears and neck (Fig. 3), until they feel hot. Lift bridge of nose with one hand seven times and do the same with other hand. Comb hair over 100 times with fingers of both hands (Figs. 4a – b) before lying down to sleep.

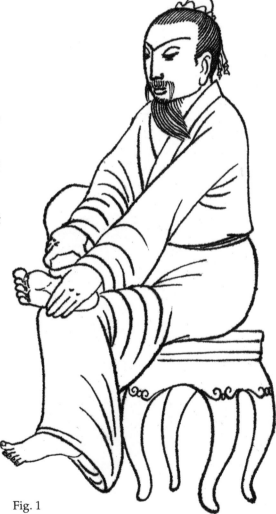

Fig. 1

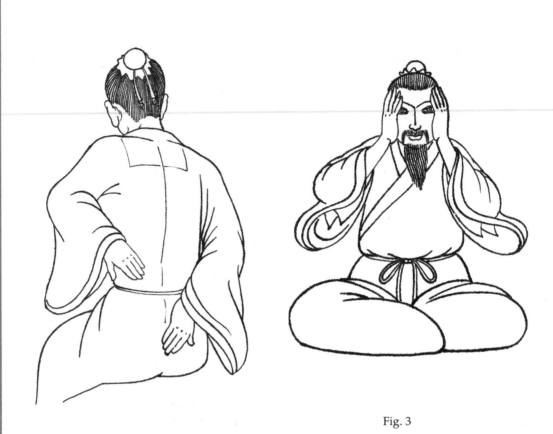

Fig. 2

Fig. 3

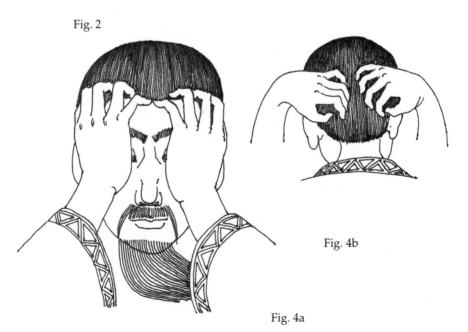

Fig. 4a

Fig. 4b

(13) Massage Eyes and Ears

Taken from *Dao Zang*, these simple self-massage exercises suit people of all ages and regular practice will improve their hearing and eyesight.

Massage ends of eyebrows 27 times with separate forefingers (Fig. 1); rub eyes and cheekbones with separate forefingers and palms (Fig. 2); work forefingers from between eyebrows up to edge of hair in 27 kneading movements (Fig. 3). Rub palms hot and massage ears in 30 rotating movements (Fig. 4). Meanwhile, touch palate with tip of tongue to produce plenty of saliva, which you swallow in any number of gulps.

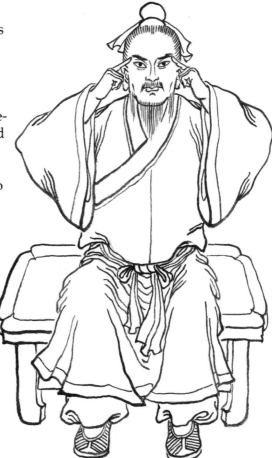

Fig. 1

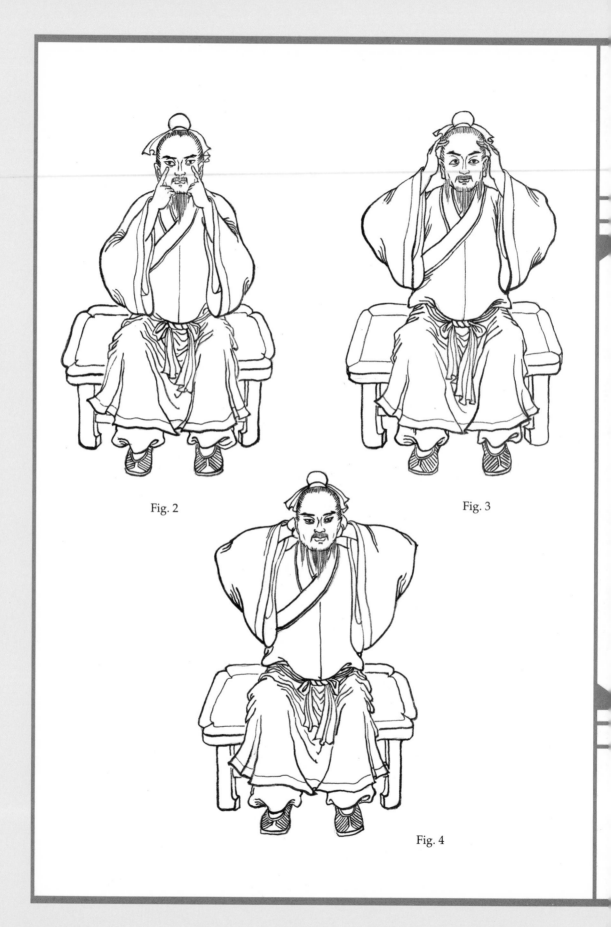

Fig. 2

Fig. 3

Fig. 4

(14) Massage for Longevity

This is taken from *Nei Gong Tu Shuo (Internal Work Illustrated)* published in 1882. It was already popular early in the 18th century.

   The last form is to be done once after repeating the other forms seven times. For beginners, however, three reps are enough in the first three days and five reps in the following four days. Practice the whole set every morning and every evening and, better yet, also at noon. It suits all age groups and both sexes — except pregnant women.

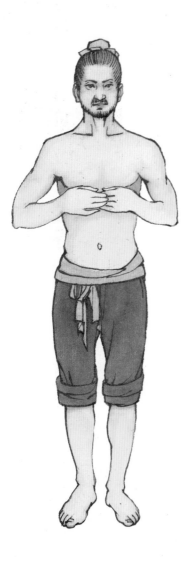

Form 1

With ring, middle and index fingers together and one hand placed on the other, massage lower part of breastbone in 21 clockwise circling movements.

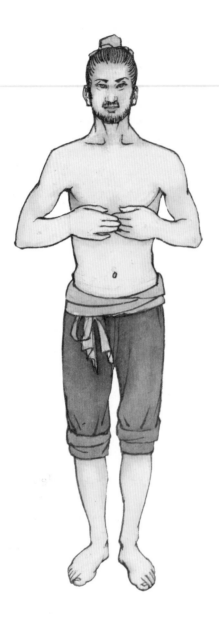

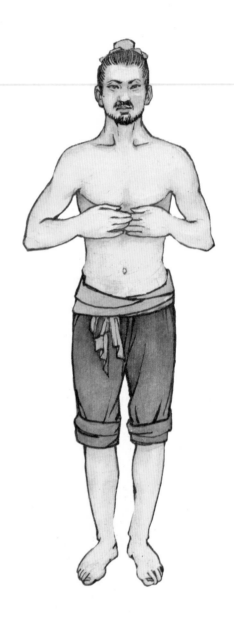

Form 2

With hands in same position, massage in kneading movements down to lower belly.

Form 3

Massage both sides of belly separately in kneading movements up to lower part of breastbone, where hands are joined.

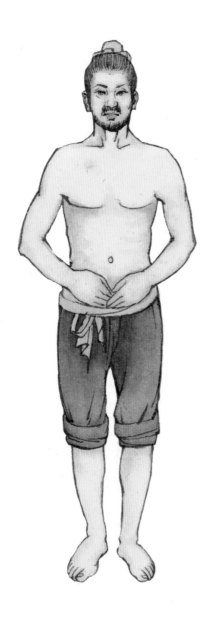

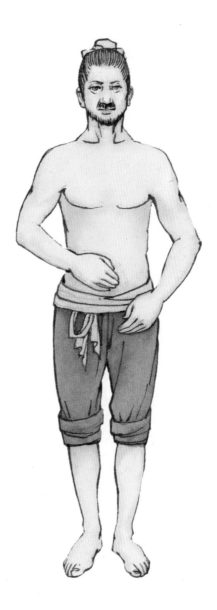

Form 4

Massage down to lower belly
21 times.

Form 5

Massage belly with right hand in
21 counterclockwise circles.

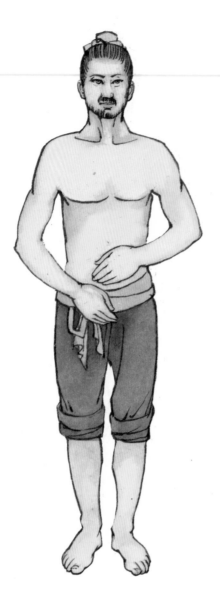

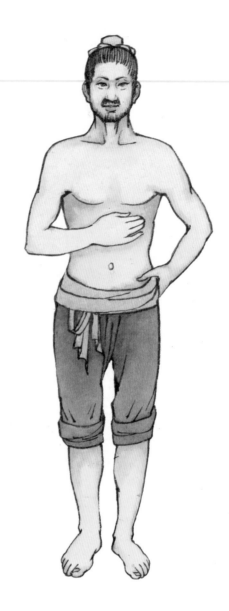

Form 6

Massage belly with left hand in 21 clockwise circles.

Form 7

With left palm holding left hip lightly, thumb in front, massage with right hand from left breast down to crotch 21 times.

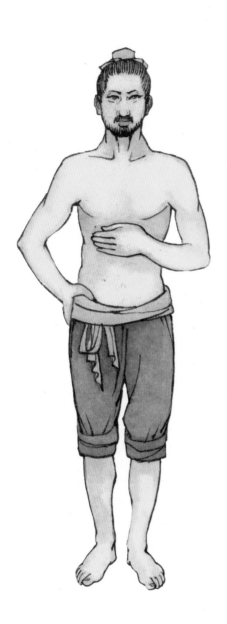

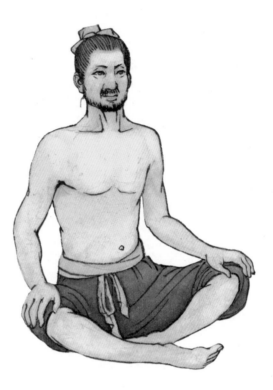

Form 9

As concluding exercise after 3, 5 or 7 reps of the preceding forms, sit down with legs crossed in front, toes slightly clenched, while both hands are placed on knees, thumb close to or away from fore-finger. Sway trunk slowly in 21 clockwise circles, so large that chest goes beyond knees.

Form 8

Do the same with right hand, starting from right breast.

(15) The Seven-Star Standing Exercises

The term "Seven Stars" refers to the Big Dipper, used for many *qigong* and *wushu* routines with seven component parts. This routine first appeared in *Can Tong Qi*, the earliest Chinese book on Taoist alchemy, written by Wei Boyang in the Eastern Han Dynasty (25 – 220). The exercises are meant to improve the circulation of *qi* and blood and maintain balance between *yin* and *yang*, as a prerequisite for good health. Movements should be soft, especially for the beginner, at a tempo that feels comfortable.

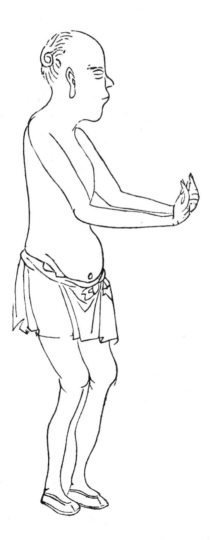

Form 1

Stand with feet about 8 inches and hands about 13 inches apart, arms bent in front, thumb and forefinger pointing up and other fingers bent, chest relaxed, shoulders dropped, trunk leaning a bit forward, and mouth and eyes closed. Keep a serene mood, with your mind's eye looking inwardly, so to speak. After a while, you'll feel yourself as soft as cotton or something floating lightly on water. Rest for a moment before doing the next exercise.

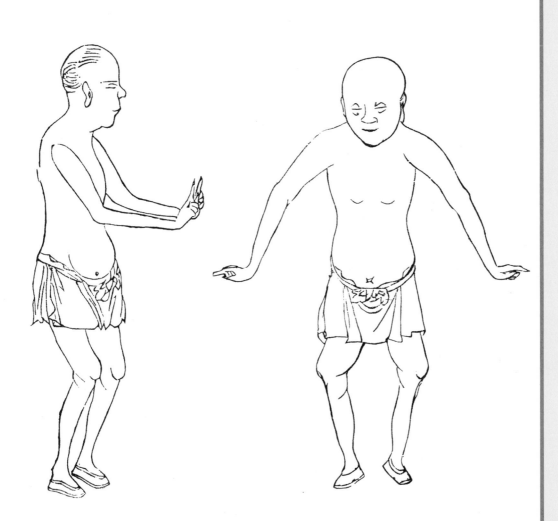

Form 2

Turn palms forward, fingertips at level with nipples. Refer to Form 1 for other particulars.

Form 3

Move hands sideways, about the width of hips from waist side, palms down and thumb and forefinger pointing outward. Stand as long as health condition permits, desirably with a sensation of pins and needles in hands.

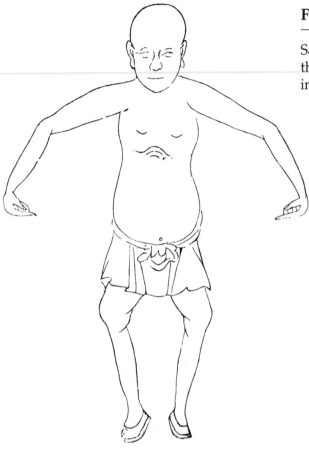

Form 4

Same as last form except that thumbs and forefingers point inward at groin level.

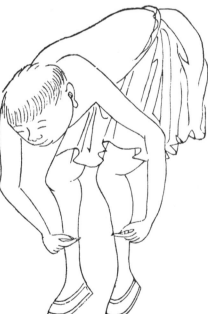

Form 5

Bend trunk forward until head is at least at waist level,* palms up and forefingers pointing at each other. Hold this position as long as befits your physical condition.

*Note: Be very careful bending over like this, especially if you have had lower back problems. Also be careful not to get dizzy. Be sure to keep knees slightly flexed. Take it slowly.

Form 6

Continuing from last form, lower both hands beside calves, palms facing back and arms hanging loosely like a rope in the well. Then unbend and bend trunk three times, with forefingers pointing down like a dart.

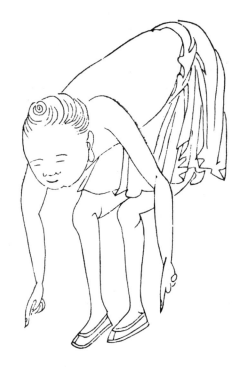

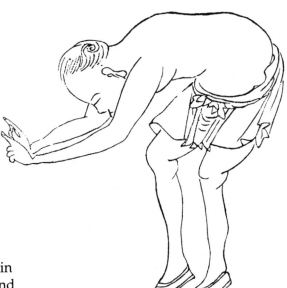

Form 7

Same as last form except that buttocks are thrown a bit backward, with hands raised in front, palms facing forward and forefingers pointing up, and, if possible, with legs fully stretched.

(16) Exercises in Eight Steps

This comes from the same origin as the "Seven-Star Standing Exercises." The movements are also the same except that hands are used alternately in four reps for either.

For Forms 1 – 2 (Figs. 1 – 2), you may start with either arm for bending and corresponding foot to take half a step forward. When alternating arms, either take a step forward with rear foot or turn body around. For Forms 3 – 7 (Figs. 3 – 7), in which feet toe the same line, only arms are alternated.

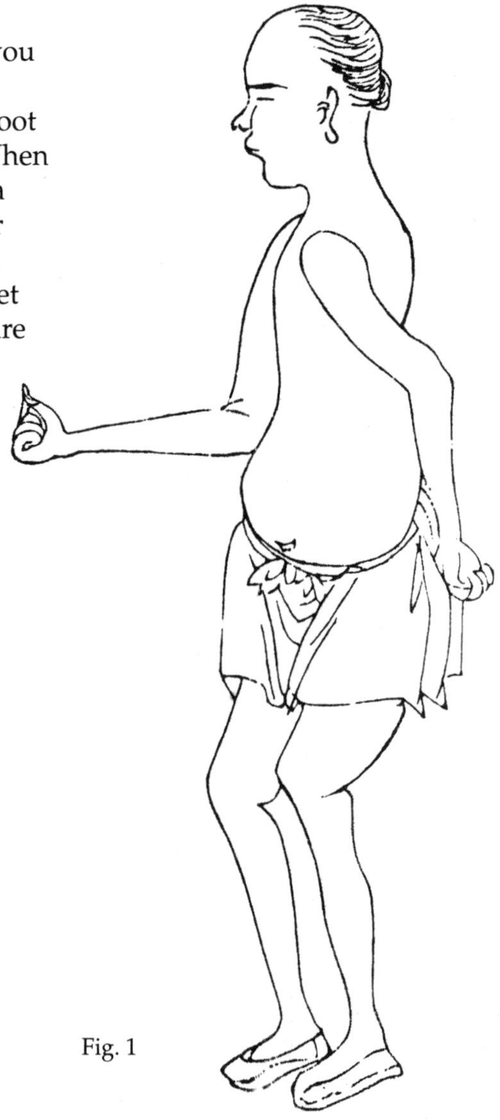

Fig. 1

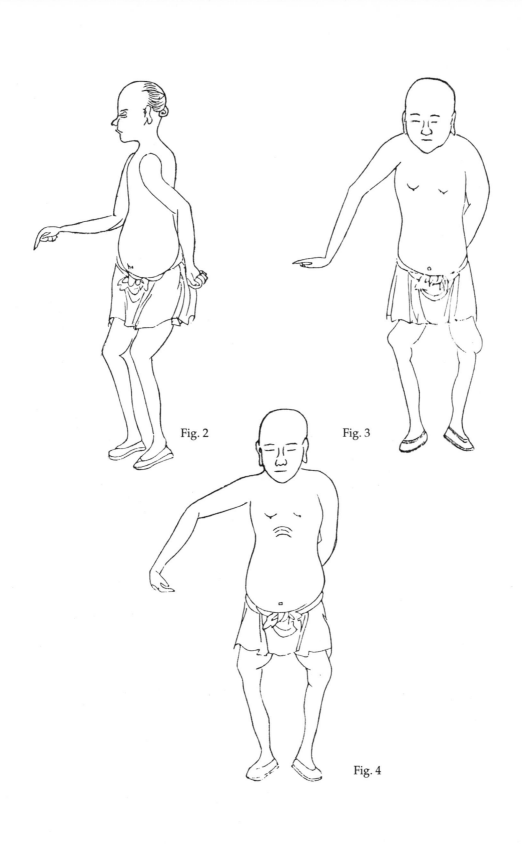

Fig. 2

Fig. 3

Fig. 4

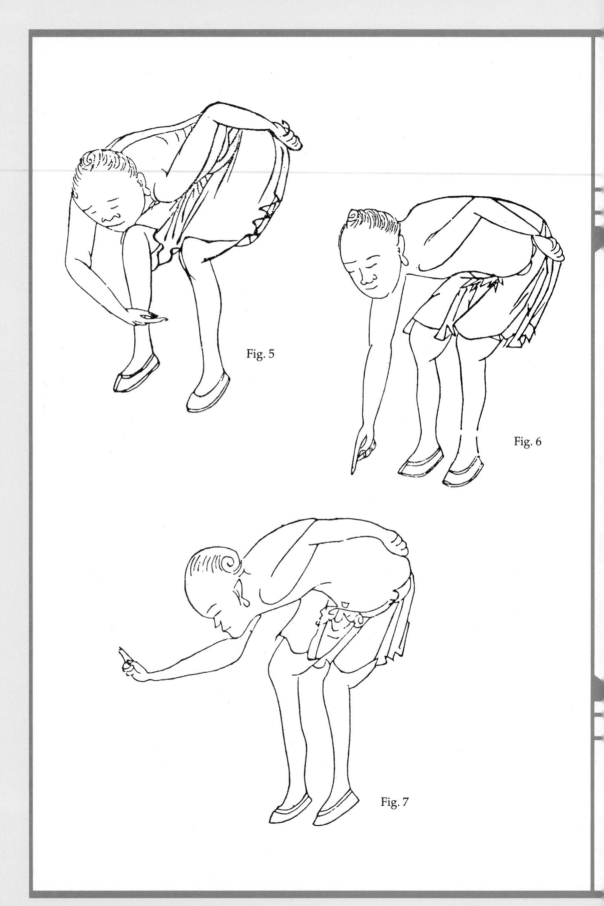

Fig. 5

Fig. 6

Fig. 7

(17) "Brocade" Exercises in Eight Forms

This is a routine of *baduanjin* exercises, which have enjoyed immense popularity among folk since ancient times. Here *ba* means "eight," *duan* means "section" and *jin* means "brocade" — a symbol of beauty. In the early 12th century, there were people "practicing *baduanjin* at midnight in imitation of the movements of the bear and the bird and by means of self-massage and regulated respiration." This kind of regimen has developed into many schools varying not only in the number of component forms, but also in movements — some in sitting and others in standing positions — yet all easy to learn for all age groups of both sexes. Today, *baduanjin* exercises are widely used for therapeutic purposes in China.

The present book contains four *baduanjin* routines: (1) in eight sitting forms; (2) in eight standing forms; (3) in four forms; and (4) in twelve forms. The first routine, dating back to the Ming Dynasty (1368 – 1644) or even earlier, is collected in *Eight Essays on Health Preserving* and *Drawings of the Heaven, Earth and Man.*

Form 1
Strike Teeth
in Deep Meditation

Sit still in deep meditation, legs crossed and hands loosely clenched. Strike upper teeth with lower teeth 36 times. Lock fingers behind head as you take nine breaths, paying a deaf ear to all sounds. Move hands to cover ears and tap back of head 24 times with middle finger pressed under index finger.

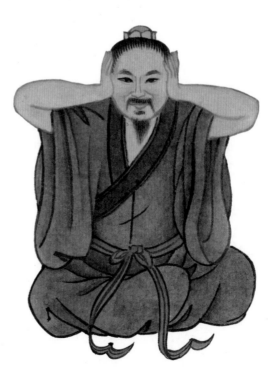

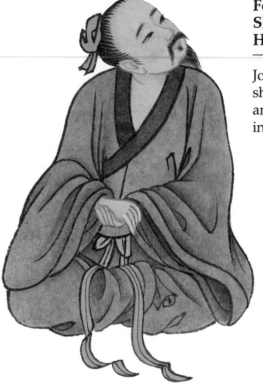

Form 2
Shake the Heavenly Pillar

Join hands in front of belly and shake head and shoulders to left and right 24 times, eyes looking in same direction.

Form 3
Gargle with Saliva

Sit upright with legs crossed and arms raised overhead. Stir tongue 36 times between hard and soft palates to produce a mouthful of saliva. Swallow it in three gulps with a gurgling sound, as if forcing something hard down throat.

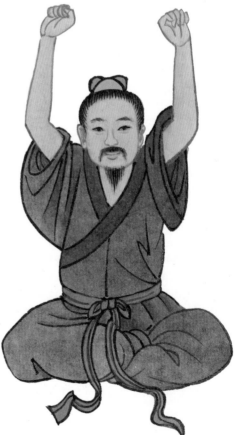

Form 4
Massage Lower Back

Hold breath and rub hands warm;
massage lower back with them 36
times and return them to front,
loosely clenched. Imagine that a
fire is spreading from heart to
lower elixir field.

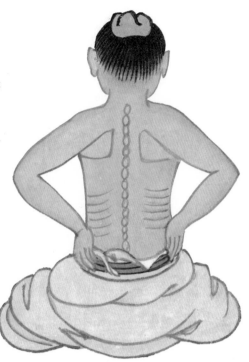

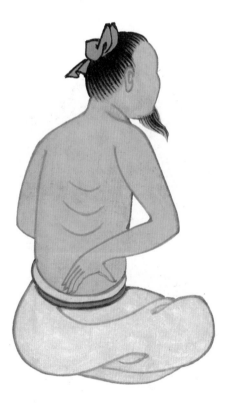

Form 5
Rotate Single
Hand on Waist Side

Rotate left shoulder 36 times with
back of right hand on lower back.
Do the same with right shoulder,
and left hand and shoulder.

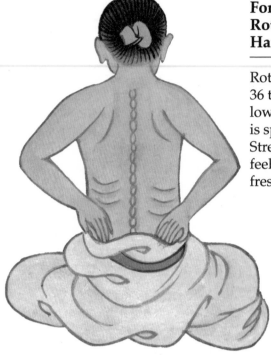

Form 6
Rotate Both
Hands on Waist Sides

Rotate shoulders simultaneously 36 times with both palms on lower back, imagining that a fire is spreading to back of head. Stretch out both legs when you feel that you've taken in sufficient fresh air through nose.

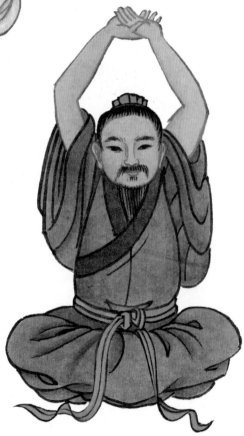

Form 7
Prop Heaven
with Both Hands

Rub hands as you breathe out air five times through opened mouth. Raise hands 3 or 9 times with fingers interlocked.

Form 8
Grasp Feet

Grasp middle part of both soles with separate hands and pull feet 12 times. Gargle mouth with saliva as you did in Form 3. Sit still with legs crossed, swallow gathered saliva in three gulps as you did in Form 3, turn head and shoulders 24 times as you did in Form 2, and rotate shoulders 24 times as you did in Form 6. Hold breath now and then as you imagine that a fire is spreading from lower elixir field to whole body.

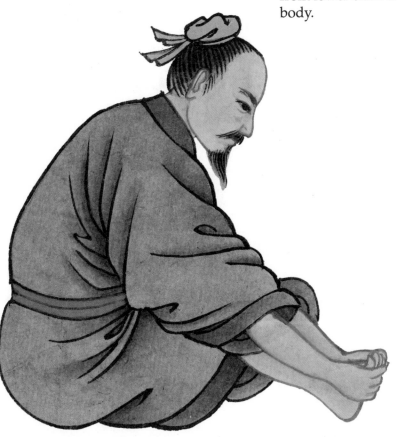

(18) "Brocade" Exercises in Eight Forms in Standing Position

Taken from *Dao Shu* compiled during the Southern Song Dynasty (1127 – 1279).

Form 1
Prop the Heaven to Improve the Functions of Triple Warmers*

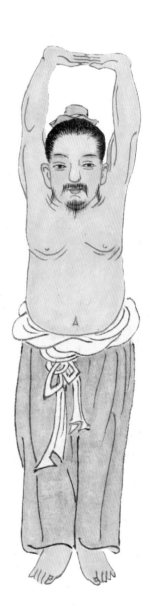

Starting position: Stand with heels together, waist and hips relaxed, chin and chest drawn in, head and back erect, armpits hollowed, shoulders dropped, arms hanging loosely at sides and fingers slightly bent. Look blankly ahead and pay a deaf ear to all sounds around. Breathe deeper with even and fine breaths.

Movements: Move hands to front of chest, palms up and five fingers held together and corresponding ones pointing at each other. With an internal rotation of arms, raise hands overhead, where they stay for one or two seconds, palms up, as if to prop up the heavens. Bring hands down sideways to original position. Seven reps.

Respiration: Inhale through nose when raising arms, with mouth half closed and tip of tongue touching palate. Exhale through mouth when bringing arms down. Breaths should be deep, long, fine and gentle.

Eyes follow both hands when they are raised overhead; then look at left hand for males and at right hand for females as they come down.

*See footnote on p. 25.

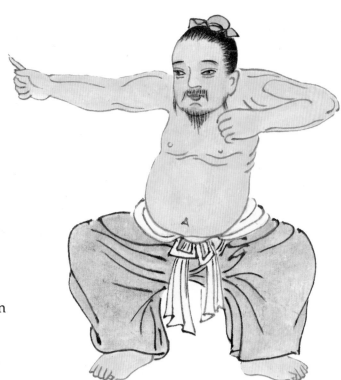

Form 2
Draw the Bow to Kill a Vulture

Starting position: Same as in Form 1 except with feet shoulder-width apart.

Movements: Raise both arms rightward slowly to shoulder level, hands loosely clenched and thumb-side up. Point up forefinger of right hand and bend left arm, elbow thrust outward and left hand in front of left shoulder, as if in an act of drawing the bow. At the same time bend both knees. After a pause of one or two seconds, straighten legs and return to starting position. Do this by reversing right and left. Seven reps.

Respiration: Inhale before you start movements, hold breath during pauses, and exhale when you put arms down.

Eyes looking over raised forefinger.

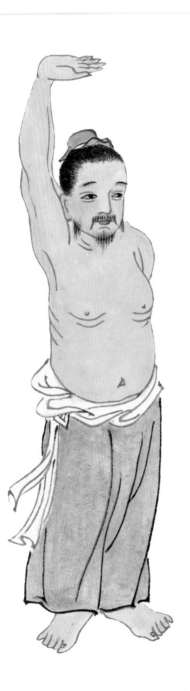

Form 3
Raise Single Arm
to Regulate the Functions
of Spleen and Stomach

Starting position: Same as in
Form 1.

Movements: Move both hands
to front of lower belly, palms up
and corresponding fingers
pointing at each other. Raise them
up to heart level. Pronate left
palm and bring it downward and
backward, while right hand, with
internal rotation of arm, is raised
overhead, palm up – both arms
stretched. After a little pause,
return hands to heart level, palms
up. Do this with hands alternated.
Seven reps. Press pronated palms
to front of lower belly and resume
starting position.

Respiration: Inhale when you
start movements, hold breath during pauses, and exhale when you
put arm down.

Eyes follow raised arm.

Form 4
Turn Head to Look
Back to Allay Five Strains*
and Seven Impairments**

Starting position: Same as in Form 1.

Movements: With arms hanging at sides and palms away from thighs, turn head and trunk slowly to right to fullest extent without leaning sideward. Pause for one or two seconds and turn to left. Seven reps.

Respiration: Inhale when you turn head and trunk sideways and exhale when you turn to front.

Eyes look ahead with turning movements.

*Referring to the strains caused by protracted use of the eyes, lying, sitting, standing and walking.

**Referring to the seven factors causing impairments by overstrain, viz., overfeeding that impairs the spleen; fury that causes adverse flow of *qi* and impairs the liver; forced overloading or prolonged sitting in damp places that injures the kidney; cold weather or drinking cold beverages that injures the lungs; sorrow and anxiety that injure the heart; wind and rain, cold and summer-heat that impair the constitution; and great shock and intemperance that impair mentality.

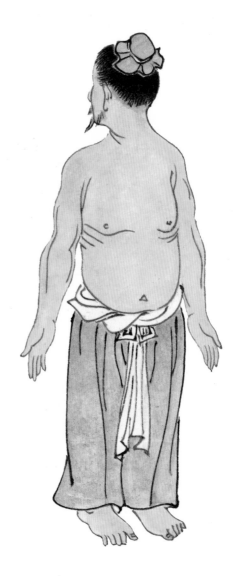

Form 5
Shake Head and
Sway Buttocks to Extinguish
Fire in Heart

Starting position: Same as in Form 2.

Movements: Lean forward and bend legs into semi-squat, palms on knees. Turn head and trunk to left and right, while swaying buttocks in opposite direction.

Respiration: Normal.

Eyes look down when you lean body forward and up when you turn it.

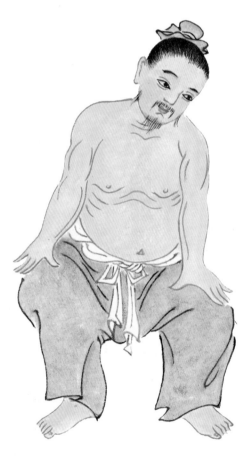

Form 6
Touch Toes to
Reinforce Kidneys

Starting position: Same as in
Form 1, except with heels about
8 inches apart.

  Movements: Raise arms
frontways and bend forward to
touch toes, or to hold heels if
possible.* Pause for one or two
seconds and straighten body,
arms stretched in front.
Seven reps.

  Respiration: Inhale through
nose when raising arms and
exhale through mouth when
bending forward. Hold breath
during pauses and inhale when
straightening body.

  Eyes follow moving hands
and look ahead with head raised
when hands touch toes or hold
heels.

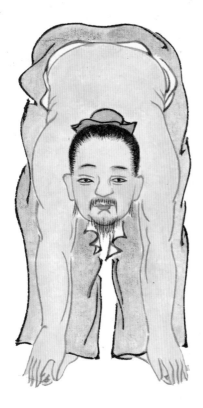

Note: Be very careful bending over like this,
especially if you have had lower back
problems. Keep your knees slightly flexed.

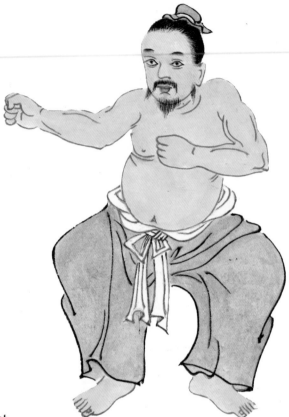

Form 7
Clench Fists and
Look Angrily to Build Up
Physical Strength

Starting position: Same as in Form 1 except with heels about length-of-foot apart and toes turned outward.

Movements: Bend legs into semi-squat and place hands, closely clenched into fists, in front of chest, knuckles down. Thrust left fist and then right fist sideways. Seven reps.

Respiration: Exhale when thrusting fist and inhale when withdrawing it.

Wide-open eyes follow moving fist.

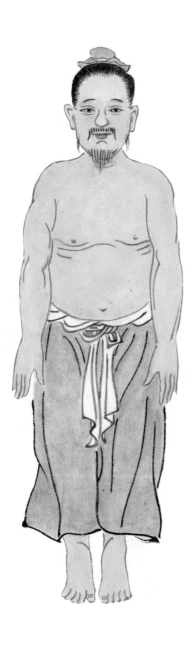

Form 8
Jolt Body to Keep
All Illnesses Away

Starting position: Same as in Form 1.

Movements: With arms hanging loosely at sides and whole body relaxed, shrug shoulders up and raise heels and then put them down to give body a jolt. 24 reps.

Respiration: Normal.

Eyes look straight ahead.

(19) "Brocade" Exercises in Four Forms

This may have been collected into *Dao Zang* (see introductory note on p. 4) during the Ming Dynasty (1368 – 1644).

Form 1
Spread Arms

Starting position: Stand erect with feet shoulder-width apart and parallel to one another, hands hanging naturally at sides, chin drawn in and eyes looking ahead. (Left)

Movements: Raise left arm frontways and right arm backward to shoulder level, palms down. (Right) Pause for a second or two before bringing arms down slowly to resume starting position. Do the same with arms alternated. Seven reps.

Respiration: Inhale through nose when raising arms and exhale through mouth when bringing them down.

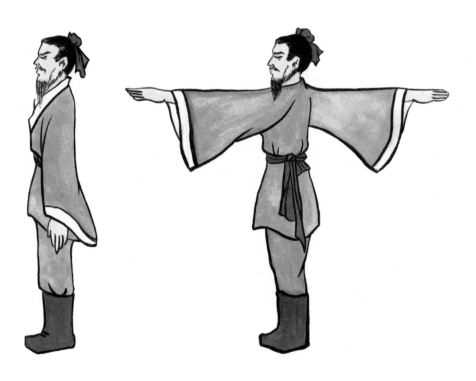

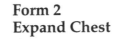

Form 2
Expand Chest

Starting position: Same as in Form 1.

    Movements: Raise both arms frontways to shoulder level and parallel to one another, hands loosely clenched and knuckles up. (Above) Move arms sideways, thumb side up. (Below) Bring arms down to resume starting position. Seven reps.

    Respiration: Inhale through nose when moving arms frontways and sideways, and exhale through mouth when bringing arms down.

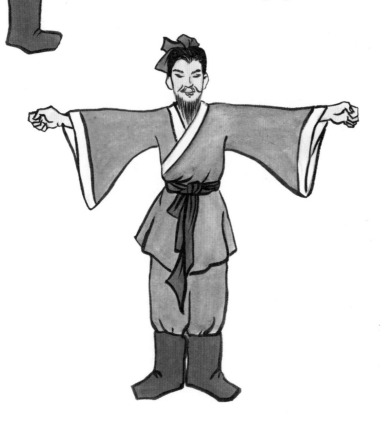

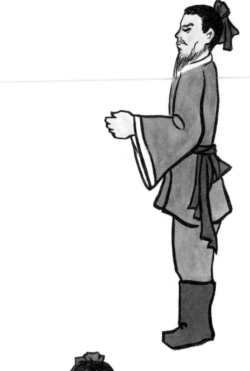

Form 3
Rotate Shoulders

Starting position: Same as in Form 1.

    Movements: Bend both arms at elbow, hands loosely clenched. Draw in chest and rotate shoulders seven times and another seven times in opposite direction.

    Respiration: Inhale when shoulders go up and exhale when they come down.

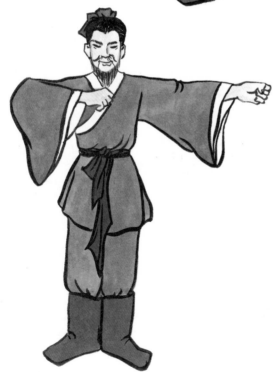

Form 4
Draw the Bow

Starting position: Same as in Form 1.

    Movements: Turn head to left as you move loosely clenched left hand to left side, arm stretched and thumb side up, while right arm is fully bent at shoulder level, elbow thrust sideways as far as possible, as if in an act of drawing the bow. Bring down arms slowly to resume starting position. Do the same with head turned to right and arms alternated. Seven reps.

    Respiration: Inhale through nose when raising arms and exhale through mouth when bringing them down.

(20) "Brocade" Exercises in Twelve Forms

This set of sitting exercises is extracted from *Can Tong Qi*, the earliest book on Taoist alchemy.

Form 1
Meditate with Eyes Closed

Sit with legs crossed in front, loosely clenched hands placed on their bends, eyes half closed, whole body relaxed and mind in perfect calm. A cushion may be placed behind. This exercise suits people of a feeble constitution.

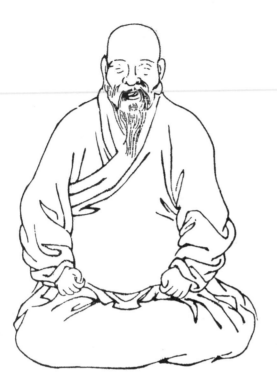

Form 2
Strike Teeth
in Deep Meditation

Sitting position as in
Form 1. Move jaws up and
down to strike lower teeth
against upper teeth 36 times
with a clicking sound. This
will help facilitate the flow
of blood in vessels and of *qi*
in *jingluo* channels.

Form 3
Drum Head
with Fingers

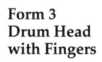

Bend trunk forward and
lower head in leg-crossed
sitting position.* Hold back
of head with both hands for
a time of nine breaths, so
gentle as not to be heard by
yourself. Cover ears with
hands and drum back of
head 24 times with middle
finger pressed under index
finger. Sit upright for a
while with hands loosely
clenched, regulating
respiration to get ready for
next exercise.

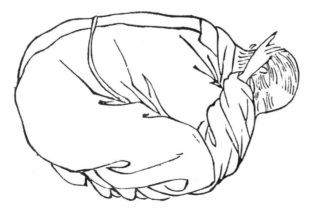

*Note: Do not lean so far forward that
you feel any pain. Proceed slowly.

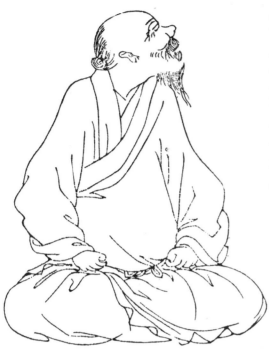

Form 4
Shake the Heavenly Pillar

With legs remaining still, turn head up slowly to left to look back, moving shoulders and arms together with head. Pause for a while and turn head to right. 24 reps. Regulate respiration and get ready for next exercise.

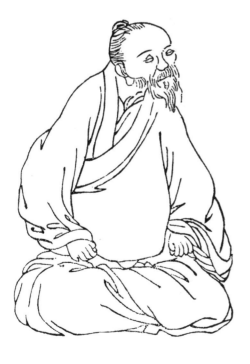

Form 5
Gargle with Saliva

Sitting position as in Form 1. Stir tongue 36 times and gargle for the same number of times with saliva, which you swallow in three gulps with a gurgling sound as though you were forcing something hard down throat.

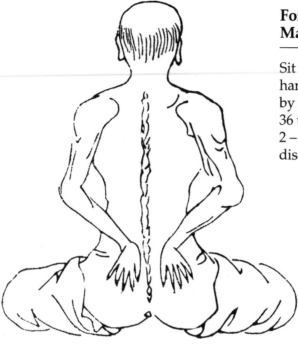

Form 6
Massage Lower Back

Sit with legs crossed and rub
hands warm. Massage lower back
by running back of hands in
36 up-and-down movements (or
2 – 4 times this many — at your
discretion).

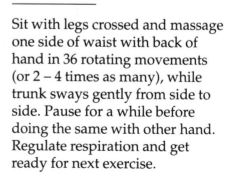

Form 7
Rotate Single
Hand on Waist Side

Sit with legs crossed and massage
one side of waist with back of
hand in 36 rotating movements
(or 2 – 4 times as many), while
trunk sways gently from side to
side. Pause for a while before
doing the same with other hand.
Regulate respiration and get
ready for next exercise.

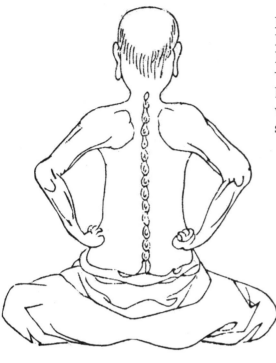

Form 8
Rotate Both
Hands on Waist Sides

Do the same as in Form 7 except with both hands moving simultaneously.

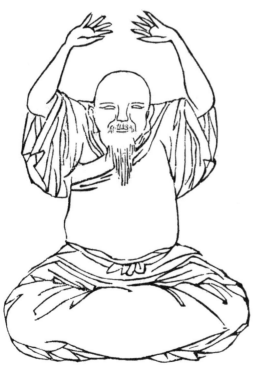

Form 9
Prop Heaven
with Both Hands

Sit with legs crossed and raise both hands overhead, palms up, for a time of three breaths (or twice or thrice as many), breathing air out through opened mouth in fine, noiseless prolonged puffs.

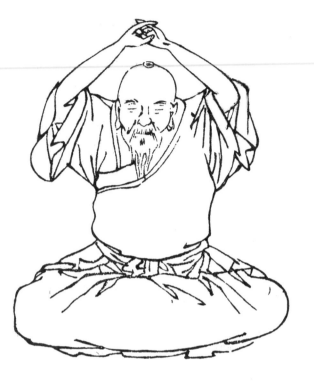

Form 10
Join Fingers Overhead

Sit with legs crossed and raise both hands overhead, fingers interlocked to press top of head three times (or twice or thrice as many). Regulate respiration and get ready for next exercise.

Form 11
Hold Toes
with Both Hands

Sit with legs stretched in front and a little apart. Bend trunk forward to grasp toes with separate hands and pull them 12 times.* Do the same with middle part of soles. Withdraw hands and sit quietly as you stir tongue to produce saliva, which you swallow after gargling. Sway trunk from side to side 12 times and rub back of hands on both sides in 36 rotating movements as you did in Form 8, imagining that a fire is burning in lower elixir field and spreading all over body.

*Note: Do not worry if you cannot reach your toes. Go only as far as is comfortable. Keep a slight flex in knees. No pain.

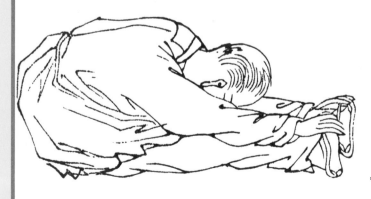

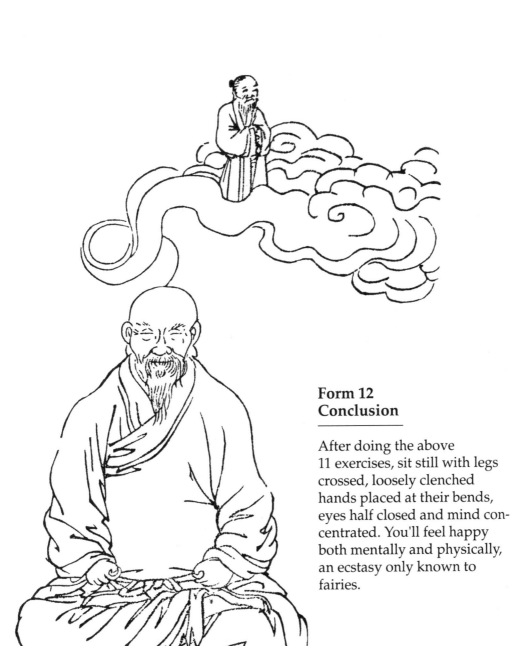

Form 12
Conclusion

After doing the above
11 exercises, sit still with legs
crossed, loosely clenched
hands placed at their bends,
eyes half closed and mind concentrated. You'll feel happy
both mentally and physically,
an ecstasy only known to
fairies.

(21) Eleven Sitting Positions

Also taken from *Can Tong Qi*. The 11 sitting positions, with legs in different postures, may be practiced at one's discretion. Each will prove its own worth in cultivating vital energy and mental faculty, promoting circulation of blood and *qi*, in improving general health condition, as long as you pay due regard to your fitness level, your proficiency in training and your pathological changes, if any.

Form 1
Easy Sitting

Sit with both legs bent naturally,* one foot behind the other, loosely clenched hands on bends of legs, thumbs bent under fingers. Keep whole body relaxed, and eyes and mouth closed while breathing through nose, and you will learn how to regulate respiration with passage of time. Pay a deaf ear to all sounds around and banish all stray thoughts and worldly worries from mind, so as to attain perfect tranquility and harmony with Nature. A long sitting will bring warmth and a slight pain or pins and needles to buttocks. Hold on as long as your health condition permits.

*See note p. 121.

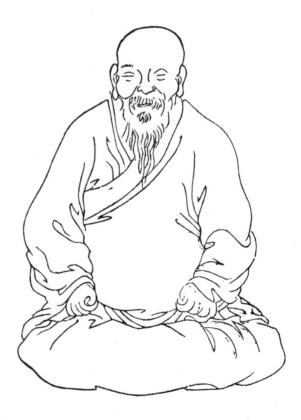

Form 2
Plain Sitting

Same as in Form 1, but with head and trunk leaning a bit forward. For those in delicate health, a soft cushion may be placed against lower back.

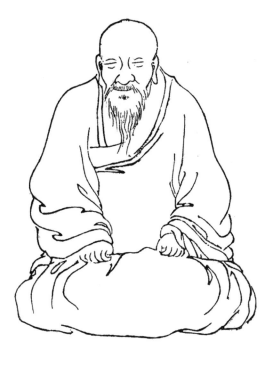

Form 3
Calm Sitting

Sit with heel of left foot against right kidney and left knee pressing right foot, and you'll feel pins and needles in heel when removed. Use legs alternately in this position.

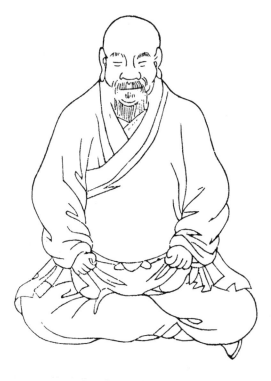

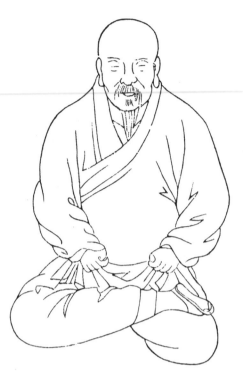

Form 4
Sitting with Legs Crossed

Sit with heel of left foot against right kidney, and right foot pressing left knee.* If you feel numbness or soreness in legs after long sitting, alternate legs in this position. At end of every sitting rub middle part of soles with hands to promote circulation of blood.

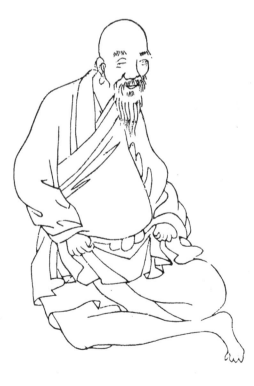

Form 5
"Fish" Sitting

Sit with one foot under coccyx and other leg stretched forward. Change legs when you feel soreness in foot. Some people may want to bear it a little longer for the benefit of circulation of blood. Don't worry about the slight pain that may appear in heel and instep and slight spasm in calf, which is indicative of the effectiveness of exercise.

*Note: The "lotus position," as shown in Forms 4, 8, 9, & 10 can cause knee problems. Most people can only achieve this position after long practice. Exercise caution.

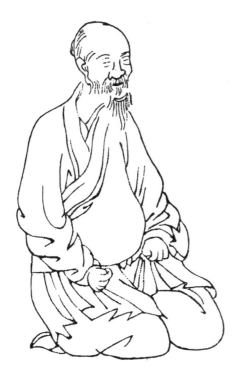

Form 6
"Spring Water" Sitting

Sit on calves, with soles turned up. You'll feel numbness in them and then, as it were, a current of "water" gushing from middle part of soles, as a result of swift circulation of blood.

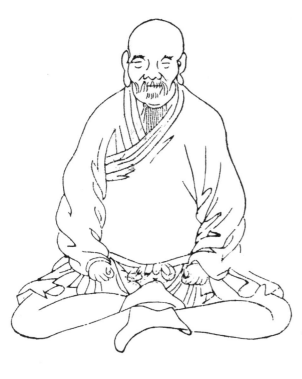

Form 7
Open-Leg Sitting

Sit with one foot in front of the other, loosely clenched hands on hips. This position greatly helps stretching of *Ren* channel* and all *jingluo* channels in buttocks. A slight soreness in hips is normal.

*Also called Front Midline channel, along which *qi* flows from pelvic cavity up to eyes.

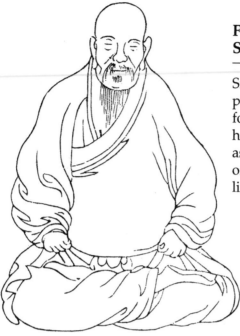

Form 8
Sitting with Feet Locked

Sit with legs crossed, left foot placed on right thigh and right foot on left thigh, loosely clenched hands on hips.* Hold on as long as possible to promote circulation of blood and *qi* through lower limbs and whole body.

Form 9
Suspended
Foot-Locked Sitting

Sit on a chair with feet locked and legs half suspended from edge of seat. As a development of the preceding form, it will produce remarkable effect through long practice.

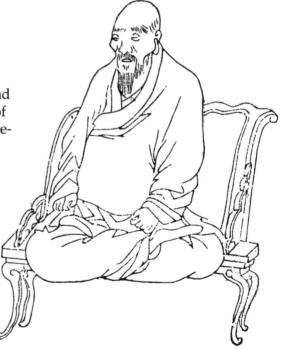

Note: This position, used in Forms 4, 9 and 10 as well, is difficult for beginners. Try it step by step.

Form 10
"To-and-Fro" Sitting

Sit on a chair with legs crossed
and suspended from edge of seat,
one foot tucked under haunches.
This position enables blood to
flow freely to and fro in vessels
and *qi* in *jingluo* channels.

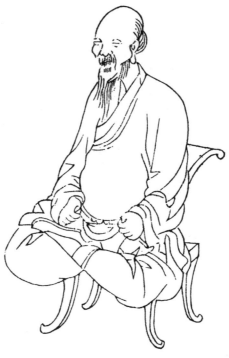

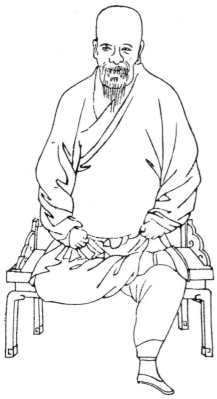

Form 11
Relaxed Sitting

Sit with left foot on floor and right
foot on left thigh, loosely clenched
hands on hips. Change legs when
you feel numbness. Regular
practice is conducive to
cultivation of *qi* and blood and
particularly suits convalescents.

(22) Exercises for Strengthening Internal Organs

Selected from *Eight Essays on Health Preserving* compiled by Gao Lian of the Ming Dynasty (1368 – 1644).

Form 1
Sitting Exercise for Strengthening the Heart

Sit upright on a stool, feet on floor and shoulder-width apart. Pound arms and body 30 times with either fist. Raise one hand overhead, palm up and fingers pointing backward, while other palm presses down, fingers pointing forward. Change hands. Eight reps, each in a gentle breath, inhaling through nose and exhaling through mouth. Hold right foot with fingers interlocked and try to stretch leg six times. Do the same with left foot. Strike upper and lower teeth 30 times, and gargle mouth with saliva before you swallow it. Long meditation with eyes closed.

As a cure for palpitation, choking sensation in chest and short breathing caused by pathogenic wind (see footnote on p. 8).

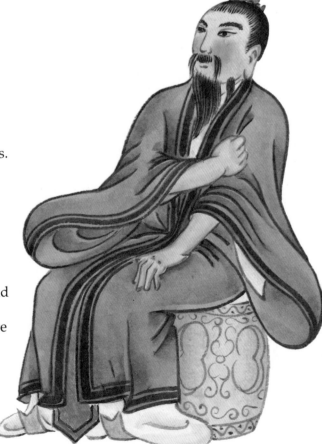

Form 2
Sitting Exercise for
Strengthening the Lungs

Sit upright on a mat with legs crossed in front. Bend trunk forward until hands touch floor. Straighten trunk and raise arms, palms up and fingers pointing backward. Three reps. Pound upper back with backs of fists 32 times and lower back another 32 times. Strike upper and lower teeth and swallow saliva. Long meditation with eyes closed.

For disorders in lungs caused by pathogenic wind.

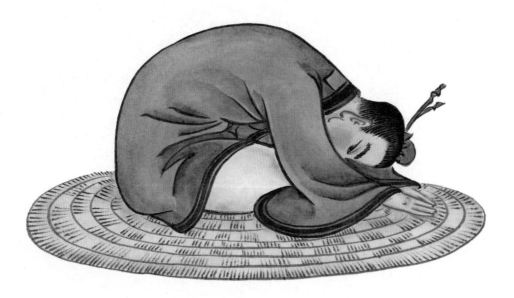

Form 3
Sitting Exercise for
Strengthening the Liver

Sit upright with legs crossed,
overlying palms on lower belly.
Turn trunk forcefully to left and
right 15 times. Join hands with
fingers interlocked and push
palms forward 7 or 8 times.

For disorders in liver caused
by pathogenic wind.

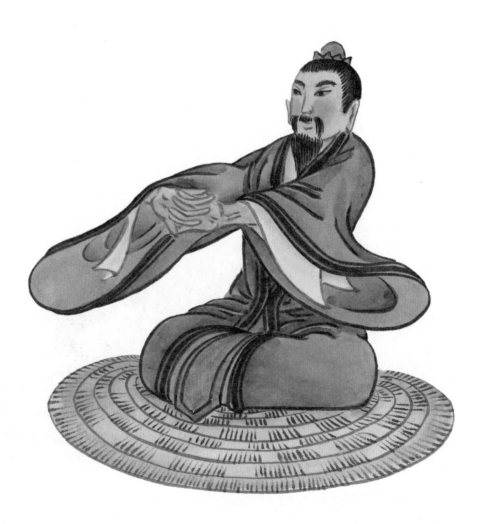

Form 4
Sitting Exercise for
Improving the Kidneys

Sit upright with legs crossed.
Place hands over ears, elbows
raised, and bend trunk rightward
and leftward 3 to 5 times. Thrust
up arms alternately 15 times.

For disorders in kidneys and
bladder.

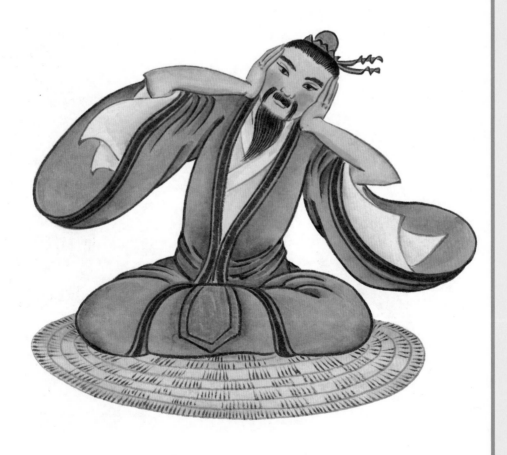

Form 5
Sitting Exercise
for Strengthening the
Gallbladder

Sit upright on a stool. Hold left foot with both hands as you sway it from side to side 15 times. Do the same with right foot.

Then with hands on stool supporting trunk from behind, throw up chest and belly to extend vertebral column. Hold this position for a moment before straightening body. 15 reps.

For disorders in gallbladder and kidneys caused by pathogenic wind.

Form 6
Sitting Exercise for
Strengthening the Spleen

Sit upright on a stool, legs
stretched out and palms
resting on knees. Raise arms,
trunk leaning backward. Hold
this position for a moment
before resuming starting
position. Three to five reps.
Then kneel in front of stool,
hands on floor at sides. Turn
head back to right and left
three to five times to look over
shoulders.

For disorders in spleen
and stomach caused by pathogenic wind and for loss of
appetite.

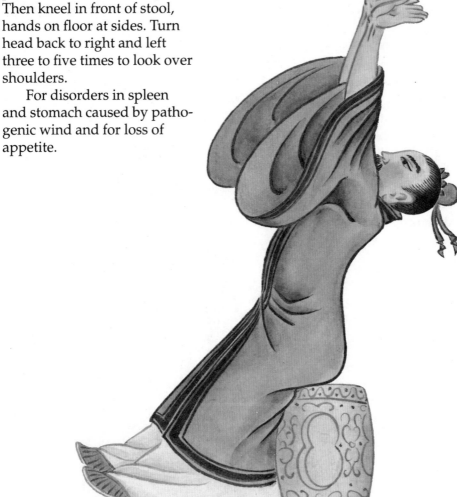

(23) Six-Sound Exercise for Health and Longevity

This set of exercises, each accompanied by a different sound in hushed voice, is selected from *Yi Men Guang Du* compiled by Zhou Lüjing, a Taoist in the Ming Dynasty (1368 – 1644). It was created by Sun Simiao (581 – 682), a renowned physician and Taoist of the Tang Dynasty. The exercises can also be done in lying and standing positions.

Form 1
"Ah" for the Heart

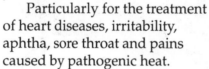

Sit upright with hands on lower elixir field, root of the tongue slightly lowered. Breathe out in a gentle, prolonged whiff through half-open mouth, uttering "ah" in a hushed voice. Breathe in through nose. As many breaths as you think fit.

   Particularly for the treatment of heart diseases, irritability, aphtha, sore throat and pains caused by pathogenic heat.

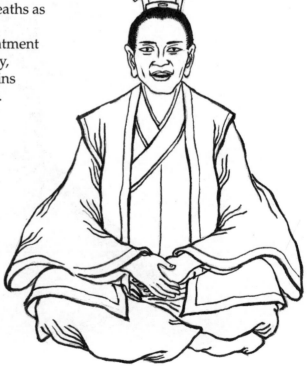

Form 2
"Chui" for the Kidneys

Hold raised knees with both
hands as you utter "chui" in a
hushed voice. Other particulars as
in Form 1.

For kidney problems and
tinnitus.

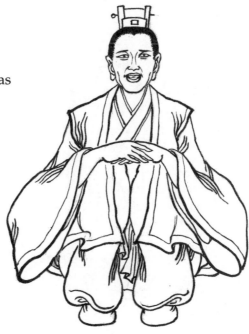

Form 3
"Hsu" for the Liver

Utter "hsu" in a hushed voice
with wide-open eyes looking
blankly ahead. Other particulars
as in Form 1.

For pains in liver and jaundiced eyes.

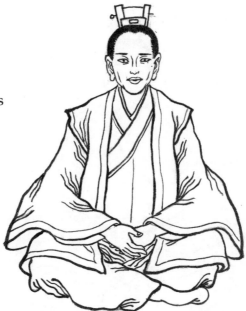

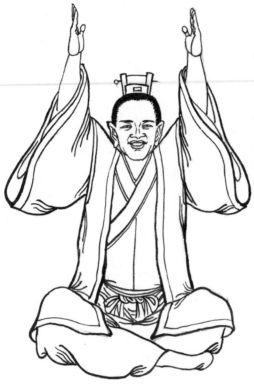

Form 4
"Si" for the Lungs

Raise both arms as you utter "si" in a hushed voice. Other particulars as in Form 1.

For disorders in lungs, choking sensation in chest, coughing, and dry throat and tongue.

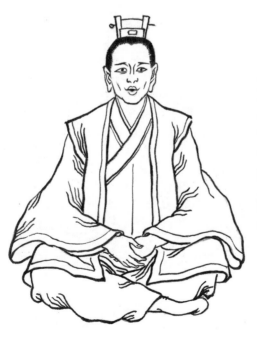

Form 5
"Hu" for the Spleen

Utter "hu" in a hushed voice with rounded lips. Other particulars as in Form 1.

For incoordination between spleen and stomach as manifested in indigestion.

Form 6
"Hsi" for the Triple Warmers

Utter "hsi" in a hushed voice with
tongue raised and corners of
mouth contracted. Other
particulars as in Form 1.

For disorders in triple warmers (see footnote on p. 25).

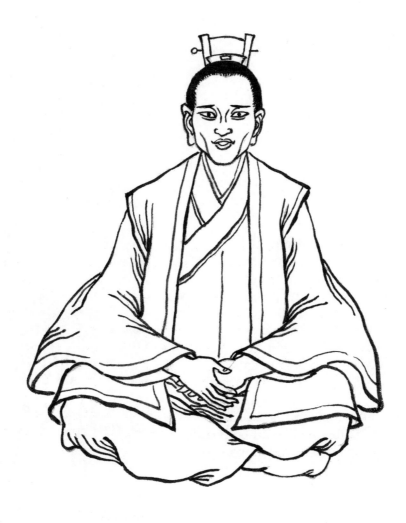

(24) Absorbing the Lunar Essence

This exercise, taken from *Yun Ji Qi Qian*, may have been in existence before the early 11th century.

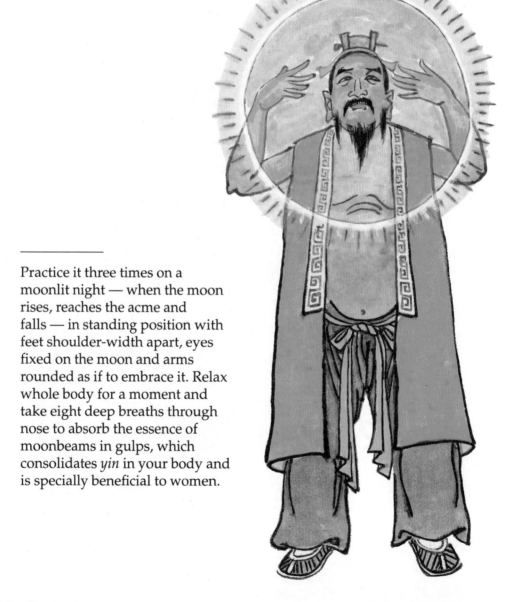

Practice it three times on a moonlit night — when the moon rises, reaches the acme and falls — in standing position with feet shoulder-width apart, eyes fixed on the moon and arms rounded as if to embrace it. Relax whole body for a moment and take eight deep breaths through nose to absorb the essence of moonbeams in gulps, which consolidates *yin* in your body and is specially beneficial to women.

(25) The Tortoise's Exercises

Also taken from *Yun Ji Qi Qian*. All the exercises are done with breath coming in and out in fine, drawn-out whiffs through the nose, which is supposed to be the breathing method used by the tortoise, a symbol of longevity in China. The length of a practice session may vary from individual to individual.

Form 1

Lie on back with both palms placed on lower elixir field and take nine gentle breaths through nose.

For treatment of nasal obstruction.

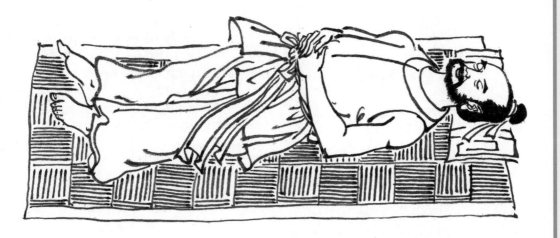

Form 2

Lie on back with head thrown back, legs bent, feet shoulder-width apart and hands on raised knees. Breathe through nose to conduct *qi* into lower elixir field.

For pains in lower back and kidneys.

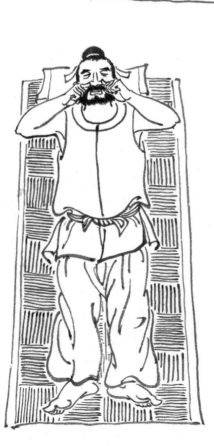

Form 3

Lie on back with legs stretched and feet shoulder-width apart. Pinch nose bridge with thumbs, conducting *qi* into upper elixir field in head.

For fatigue and imbalance between *yin* and *yang*.

Form 4

Lie on back with left hand grasping hair and right hand holding nape of neck, as you breathe gently through nose.

This exercise keeps *yin* and *yang* in balance and promotes circulation of *qi* and blood.

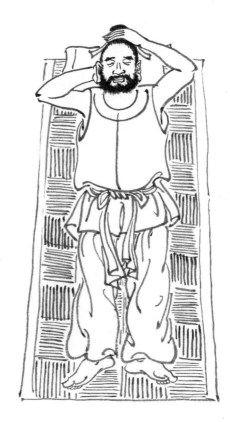

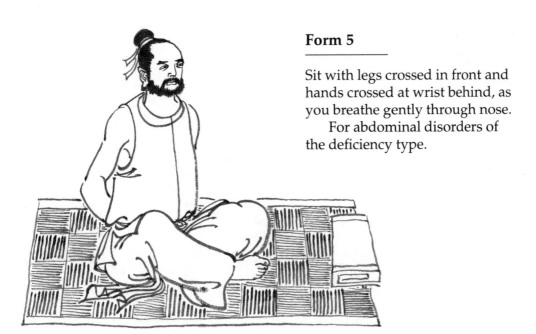

Form 5

Sit with legs crossed in front and hands crossed at wrist behind, as you breathe gently through nose.

For abdominal disorders of the deficiency type.

Form 6

Fall back in sitting position. With hands akimbo and feet raised as high as possible, breathe gently through nose.

For lack of concentration and nausea.

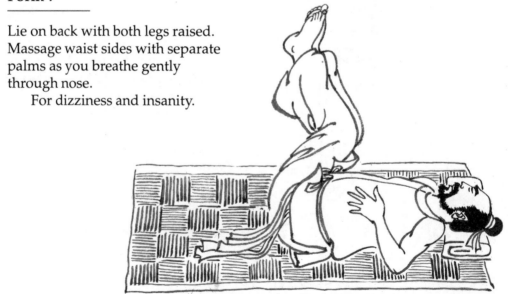

Form 7

Lie on back with both legs raised. Massage waist sides with separate palms as you breathe gently through nose.

For dizziness and insanity.

Form 8

Lie on back with one hand
holding both feet and other hand
raised as if holding a rope.
     For stubborn piles.

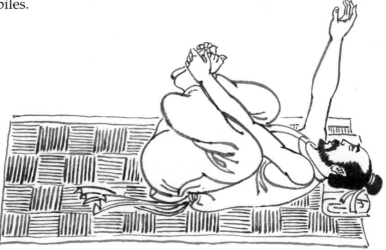

Form 9

Sit with legs stretched in front.
Pull feet with separate hands.
     This exercise improves
function of intestines and stops
vomiting.

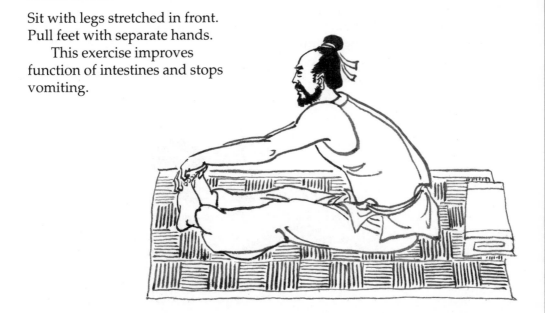

Form 10

Sit facing east, with both palms on lower elixir field and head thrown back. Take five deep breaths as you stir up saliva and swallow it.

For thirst and bitterness in mouth.

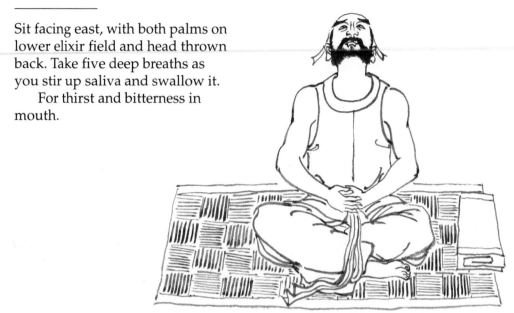

Form 11

Sit with legs crossed or one placed before the other, arms folded and head lowered. Bend trunk forward 12 times, holding breath when trunk is bent and breathing through nose when trunk is unbent.

For indigestion.

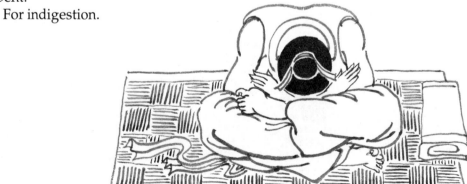

Form 12

Sit with legs crossed, palms on lower elixir field. Lower head 12 times, holding breath before it is raised.

For scabies and skin ulcers.

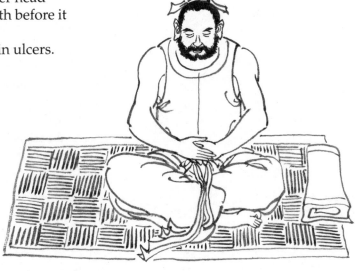

Form 13

Sit with legs crossed and hands on nape of neck, fingers interlocked, as you breathe through nose.

For disorders caused by various pathogens.

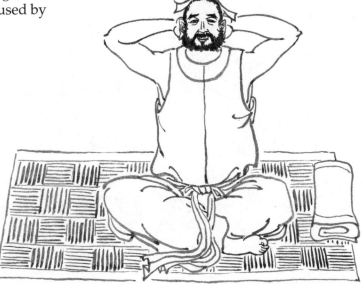

(26) The Frog's Exercises

Also taken from *Yun Ji Qi Qian*.

Form 1

Sit with legs crossed and arms bent at elbow. Swing one arm forward and the other backward 12 times, and then both together from side to side another 12 times.

For overstrain and edema.

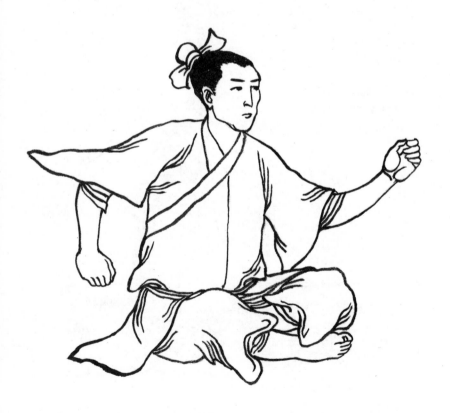

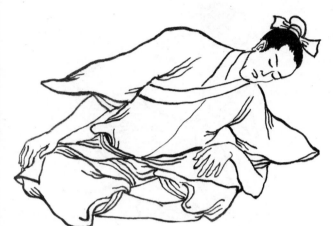

Form 2

Sit upright with legs crossed,
palms on separate knees. Bend
trunk leftward as you exhale
through nose. After a little
pause, return to upright
position as you inhale. Then
bend trunk rightward. 12 reps.
    For clearing sputum.

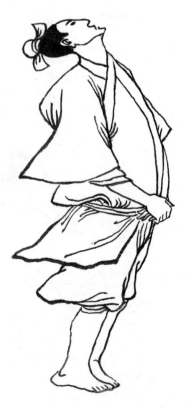

Form 3

Take nine breaths three times a
day — at sunrise, noon and
sunset — facing the sun in
standing position, with feet
shoulder-width apart, so as to
absorb the essence of sunshine.
    To strengthen *yang* in body.

Form 4

Stand with trunk leaning forward
and legs bent in semi-squat, palms
between thighs and toes
purchasing ground, as you
breathe through nose.

    To strengthen waist and
kidneys.

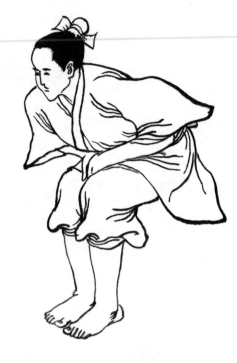

Form 5

Sit with feet held in hands, fingers
interlocked. Pull hands many
times against a resisting force
from feet.

    For seminal emission.

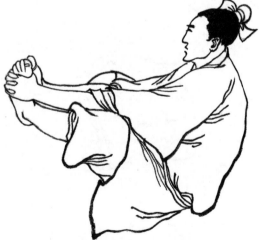

Form 6

Sit with legs bent and arms
extended in front. Pull down
thumb of left hand and then of
right hand.
    For aching joints.

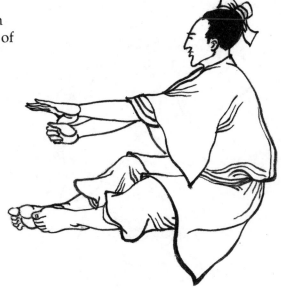

Form 7

Sit quietly with legs bent and
hands pressing toes.
    For aching lower back causing
inability to turn and bend trunk.

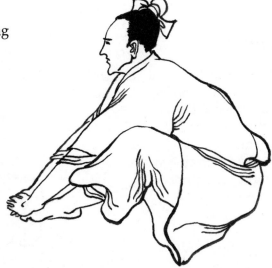

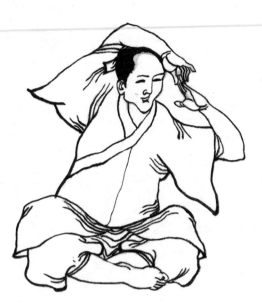

Form 8

Sit with legs crossed and right arm bent overhead to hold fingers of left hand as the latter pulls down. Change hands. As many reps as you see fit.

For stiffness in neck.

Form 9

Sit with legs crossed, left arm bent across chest and right hand on left shoulder. Bend trunk leftward and then rightward after a short pause, breathing through nose.

For pains in waist and knees and urethrophraxis.

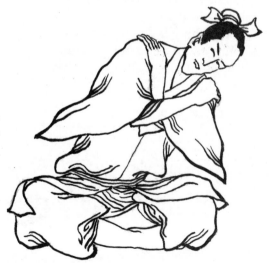

(27) *Yijinjing:* Limbering-Up Exercises for Tendons and Muscles

Yijinjing has existed for centuries as a favorite with the populace and is still widely used in sanatoriums and hospitals for therapeutic purposes. Two ancient routines are selected into this book, one from Chen Yi's *A Collection of Annals* published in the Ming Dynasty (1368 – 1644), with titles given later for the 12 forms, and the other (p. 169) from *Internal Work Illustrated*, published in 1882.

There are different views regarding the origin of *yijinjing*. Some people have attributed it, without sufficient authenticity, to Bodhidharma (? – 528 or 536), an Indian abbot who preached Buddhism in China and founded the Zen sect.

Form 1
Working at a Mortar

Stand still for a while with arms hanging loosely at sides, eyes looking ahead and mind concentrated on lower elixir field. Move hands to front of lower belly and then up to shoulder level as if they were holding something heavy. After a short pause, swing hands down to waist sides. 21 reps. Imagine that you are working with a pestle to unhusk grains in a mortar.

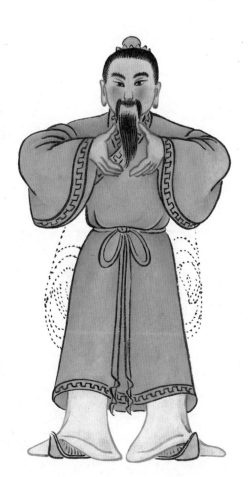

Form 2
Carrying the Grain
with a Shoulder Pole

Stand as in Form 1. Raise arms
sideways to shoulder level, fingers
held together and pointing up; put
them down slowly to waist sides
after a short pause. Then raise left
arm forward and right arm
backward, both to shoulder level
and put them down slowly at
waist sides after a short pause. Do
the same with arms alternated.
Seven reps. Imagine that you are
carrying two buckets of grain on a
shoulder pole, one arm on its front
part and the other on its rear part.

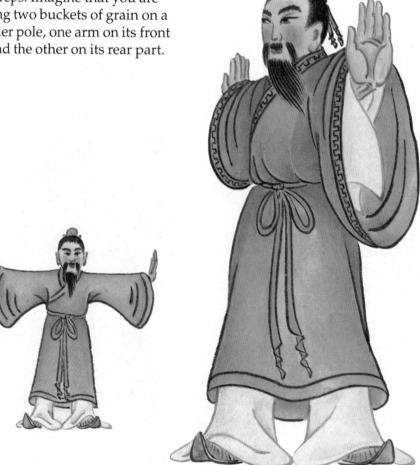

Form 3
Winnowing Grains

Stand as in Form 1. Bend trunk
forward and hollow palms,
corresponding fingers pointing at
each other, as if they were holding
something heavy. Raise both
hands overhead with an internal
rotation of arms, palms up and
corresponding fingers pointing at
each other. Put down hands after a
short pause. Seven reps. Imagine
that you are picking up a winnow-
ing pan and raising it overhead to
scatter the chaff to the wind.

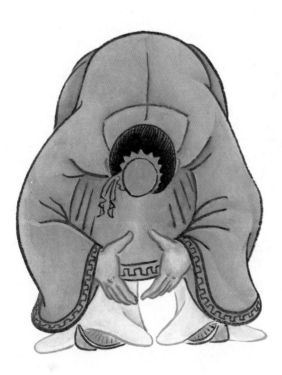

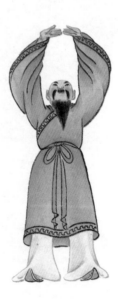

Form 4
Shifting a Bag of
Grain on Shoulders

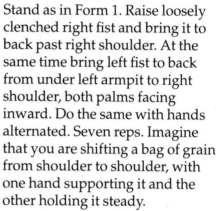

Stand as in Form 1. Raise loosely clenched right fist and bring it to back past right shoulder. At the same time bring left fist to back from under left armpit to right shoulder, both palms facing inward. Do the same with hands alternated. Seven reps. Imagine that you are shifting a bag of grain from shoulder to shoulder, with one hand supporting it and the other holding it steady.

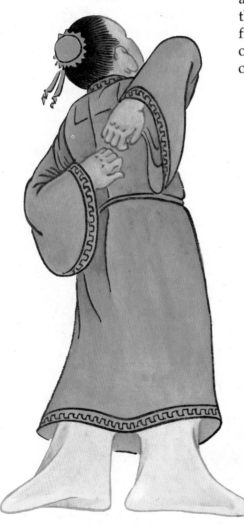

Form 5
Piling Up Grain Bags

Squat down with feet shoulder-width apart and hands above knees, palms up and corresponding fingers pointing at each other. Stand up on feet as you stretch out both arms in front of chest, palms facing forward and fingers pointing up. Then move arms sideways as you squat down for another arm hold. Seven reps. Imagine that you are piling up bags of grain.

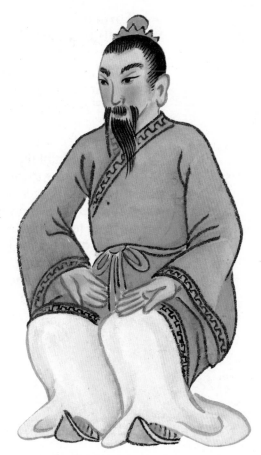

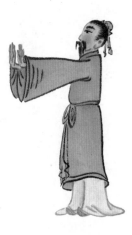

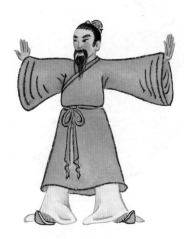

Form 6
Pulling a Cart

With body turning to right, take a
forward step in same direction
with right foot to form a right
"bow stance," with front leg bent
and rear leg stretched. At the same
time raise right fist in front of face,
elbow thrust forward, while left
fist moves down to left, elbow at
shoulder level and forearm
vertical to ground. After a short
pause, do the same in a right bow
stance by reversing right and left.
Seven reps. Imagine that you are
pulling a cart with a rope over
shoulders.

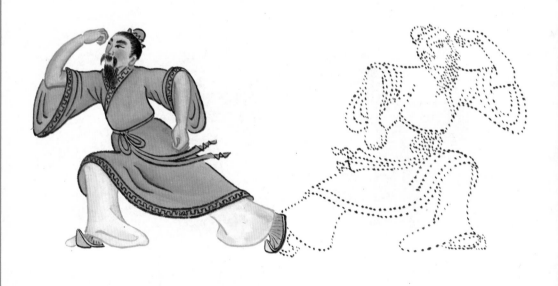

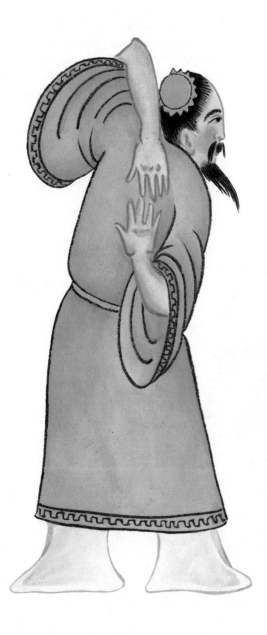

Form 7
Tugging a Boat

Stand with feet shoulder-width apart. With head turning to right, touch spinal column with both hands — left coming from over left shoulder and right from under right armpit with an internal rotation of both arms. Now left palm is facing inward and right palm outward. After a short pause, do the same with hands alternated. Seven reps. Imagine that you are tugging a boat with a rope on back.

Form 8
Loading and
Unloading the Grain

Stand with feet shoulder-width apart and squat down to form a "horse-riding stance." Bend both arms at right angle, elbows at waist sides and palms facing forward. Supinate both palms as if they were holding something in front of navel. After a short pause, pronate palms as you stand upright, arms hanging at sides. Seven reps. Imagine that you are loading and unloading something heavy.

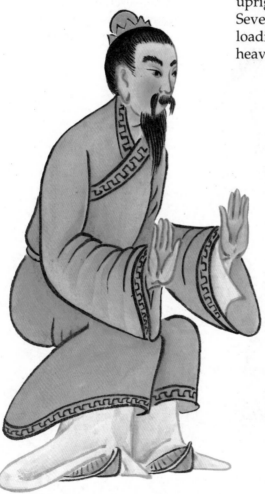

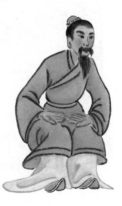

Form 9
Stacking Up the Grain

Stand upright with feet shoulder-width apart. Place left fist on left part of belly, knuckles down. Bend forward to left as you reach out right hand, hooked, in same direction. Stand upright, arms hanging at sides, and do the same by reversing right and left. Seven reps. Imagine that you are bending over a silo-like stack to put grain into it.

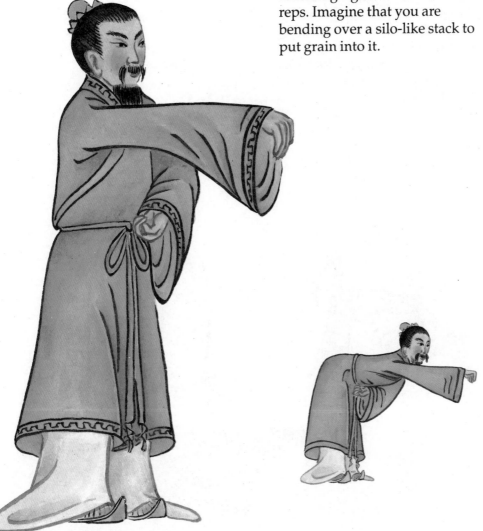

Form 10
Protecting the Grain

Stand with feet shoulder-width apart. With trunk turning to left, take a forward stride in same direction with left foot to form a left bow stance. Place both palms on floor before front leg, head raised. After a short pause, with trunk turning to right, withdraw left foot to resume straight body position. Do the same in a right bow stance by reversing right and left. Seven reps. Imagine that you are protecting something on the ground.

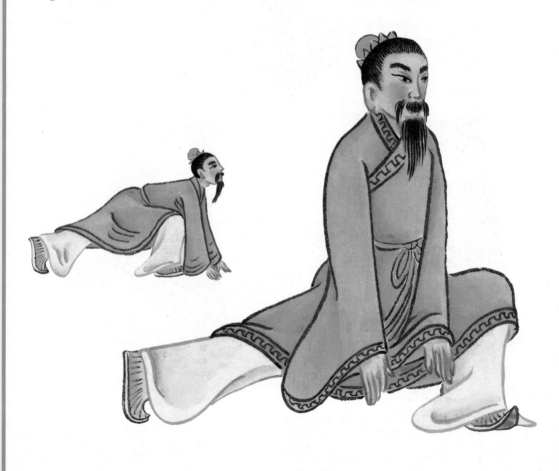

Form 11
Garnering Grains

Stand upright with feet shoulder-width apart. Hold nape with both hands and bend forward to touch floor with hands. Then straighten body, arms hanging at sides.
14 reps. Imagine that you are picking up something on the ground.

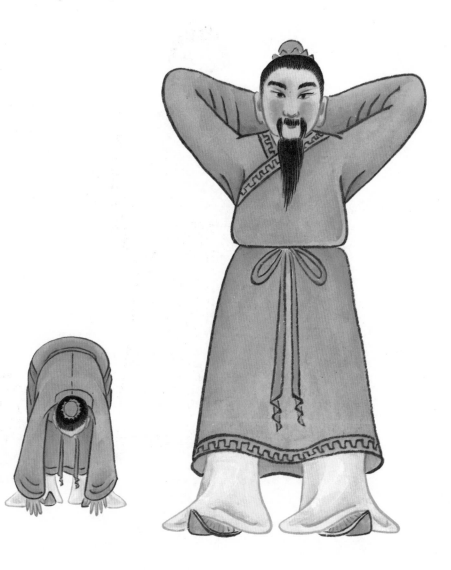

Form 12
Storing the Grain

Stand upright with feet shoulder-width apart. Stretch arms frontways and sideways, palms down. Squat down as you press palms down to front of shins where they are supinated. Stand up and move arms frontways and sideways at shoulder level, palms pronated. Put arms down at sides. From 7 to 14 reps. Imagine that you are picking up something for storage.

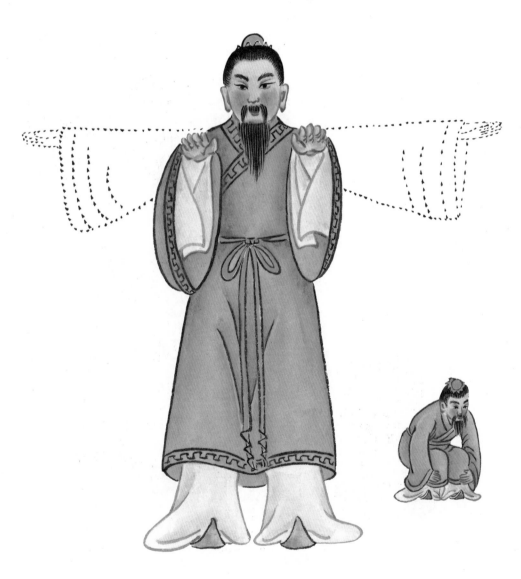

(28) *Yijinjing* Exercises in Twelve Forms

See introductory note on p. 157.

Starting Position

Stand erect with feet shoulder-
width apart, toes turned outward,
arms hanging naturally at sides,
hands pressed against thighs, chin
drawn in and eyes half closed.
Keep whole body relaxed and
mind concentrated as you take
three deep breaths.

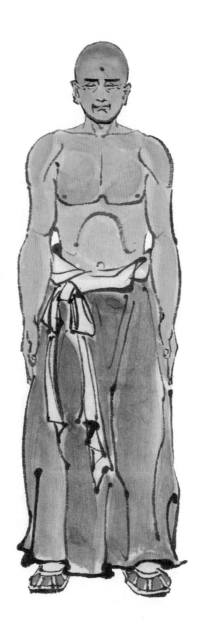

Form 1
General Skanda
Holds the Cudgel

Stand upright with heels together. Raise arms frontways to shoulder level, palms facing each other. Breathe in as you bend arms at right angle. Breathe out as you join palms in front of chest. Imagine that *qi* is flowing from four limbs into middle elixir field (xiphoid). Pause for a minute at end of exercise.

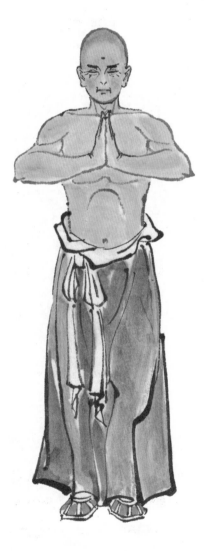

Form 2
Shoulder Up
the Evil-Subduing Cudgel

Continuing from last form, separate palms as you drop them slowly to front of lower elixir field and, after a short pause, further down until arms are fully stretched; then separate hands and raise arms sideways to shoulder level, palms down and heels off floor.

Sink *qi* to lower elixir field when lowering arms and conduct it to palms when raising arms sideways. Breathe naturally in a calm state of mind. Pause for a minute at end of exercise.

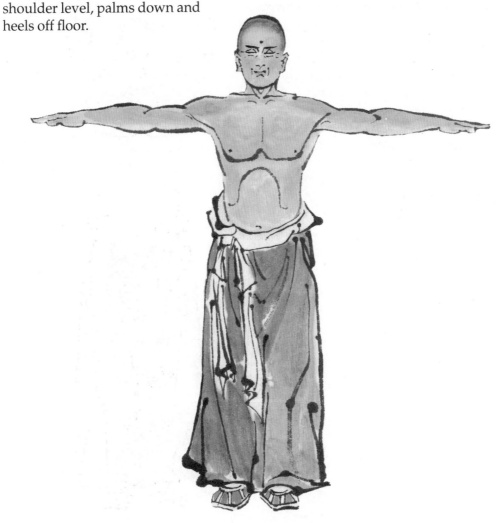

Form 3
Prop Heaven with Palms

Continuing from last form, raise arms slowly overhead, palms turned up, corresponding fingers pointing at each other and heels raised, as if you were lifting something heavy. At the same time, with tongue touching palate, strike lower teeth against upper teeth to produce saliva, which you swallow — supposedly into lower elixir field. Then turn heels outward and put them down while arms are lowered slowly sideways to shoulder level, with fingers bent one after another (starting with little finger) to turn hands into loosely clenched fists. Inhale when raising arms and hold breath for a while or breathe normally when hands stay overhead. Pause for half a minute at end of exercise.

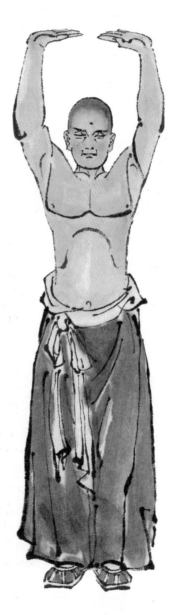

Form 4
Gather the Big Dipper

Continuing from last form, lower left arm to back in an arc and press palm forcibly downward, while right hand is raised overhead, palm down. At the same time turn head to right to look up at right hand and raise right heel to form a right "T step," with bulk of body weight on left leg. Pause for half a minute as you take 3 – 5 deep breaths (left). Repeat these movements by reversing right and left (right).

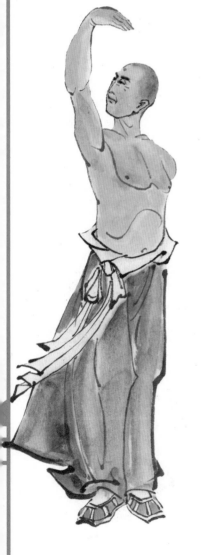

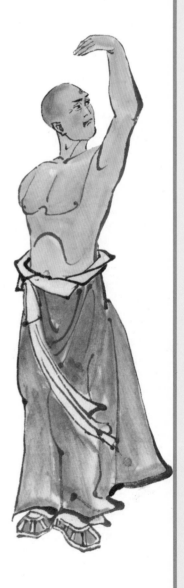

Form 5
Drag Nine Oxen by Tail

Continuing from last form, move left hand to side of left hip, fingers bent and palm down. At the same time raise right hand to shoulder level, bend arm at elbow, hand turned into hollow fist and body leaning to right at an angle of 45°. Then turn to right and take a forward step in same direction to form a right bow stance with rear leg stretched and front leg bent at knee, which does not go beyond toes, as if you were pulling a cart with a long rope over shoulders (left). Turn about on right foot and take a forward step with left foot. Repeat these movements by reversing right and left (right).

Breathe naturally and concentrate mind on palms.

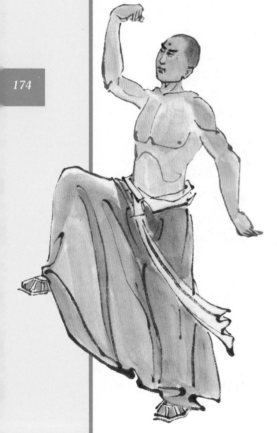

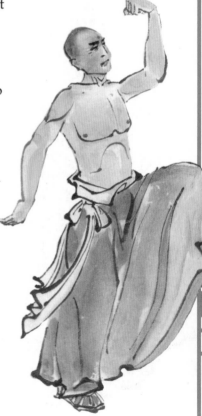

Form 6
Show Claws and Flash Wings

Continuing from last form, stamp ground and take a step forward with right foot to place it beside left foot and stand upright. Withdraw fists to waist sides, knuckles down. Then open palms and push them forward seven times, fingertips at shoulder level — fingers slightly spread out when hands are withdrawn to waist sides for next push. Imagine that you are opening a window to look at the moon when you push palms forward and that a tide is coming in when you withdraw hands to waist sides.

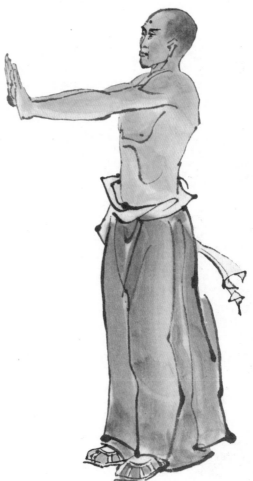

Form 7
Nine Ghosts
Unsheathe Their Sabres

Continuing from last form, raise arms sideways to shoulder level, palms up. Then bend trunk a bit forward and cock head slightly on left side as you move right hand to back of head, tips of middle and index fingers pinching left ear lobe and pulling it gently to right. At the same time, with trunk turning to left, move left arm behind, back of hand pressed on spinal column and running up it, fingers pointing up. Bend legs slightly and lower head to look down at instep of right foot (left).

Stand upright again and repeat above movements by reversing right and left (right). Stand still for half a minute at end of exercise.

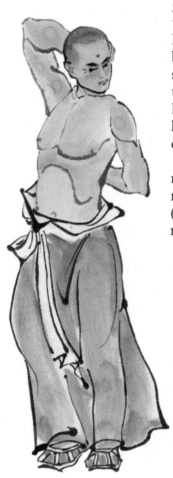

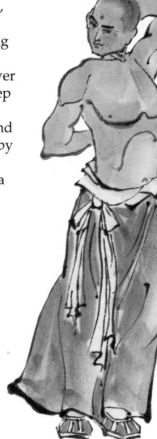

Form 8
Body Rises and Falls

Continuing from last form, take a side step with left foot, both feet turned outward. Raise arms sideways to shoulder level, palms down. Bend legs at knee to form a "horse-riding stance" as you press palms down to knee level. Straighten legs slowly to stand upright as you raise arms up to shoulder level, palms supinated. Three or five reps.

Inhale when pressing palms down as if you were forcing a floating log into water, and exhale when raising arms as if you were lifting something heavy.

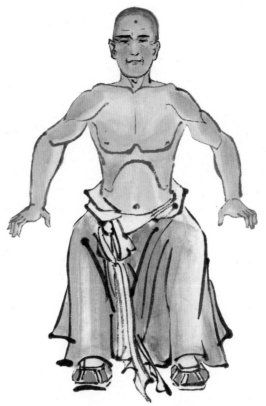

Form 9
The Black Dragon Pushes Its Claws

Continuing from last form, place left foot beside right foot to stand upright, hands shaped like claws. Lower left hand to waist side and, with trunk turning to left, thrust right hand to front, with arm slightly bent at elbow and waist and belly relaxed. Withdraw right hand to waist side for two more thrusts, first obliquely and second directly to left (above). Turn about on left with a jerk of head, a searching glance in eyes. Repeat thrusts with left hand (below).

Inhale when withdrawing hand and exhale when pushing it, each time accompanied by a hushed "shoo." Every push and pull should be accentuated by a slight body turn.

Form 10
The Tiger
Pounces on Its Prey

Continuing from last form, place left hand in front of belly and with body turning to right and bending forward, take a stride forward with right foot as you thrust both palms downward in an arc — like a tiger pouncing on its prey. Now you are in a right bow stance, both palms on floor and head raised to look to right and left (above). Then, with hands supporting body, bend left leg at right angle, lift left foot with sole facing upward and push body up three to five times. With palms off floor and supinated, turn about on left; pronate palms for another pouncing movement, reversing right and left (below).

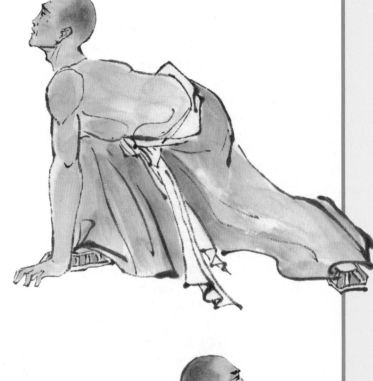

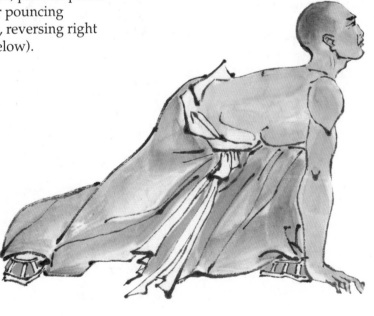

Form 11
Beat Drum and Bend Trunk

Continuing from last form, put
down right foot, raise trunk and
turn to right, moving right foot
half a step toward left foot, so that
they are about shoulder-width
apart and you are in squatting
position. Raise both hands to back
of head, palms covering ears.
With whole body relaxed, tap
back of head with hands
alternately, seven times for
either — with ring, middle and
index fingers slightly bent, in a
percussion massage known as
"beating the heavenly drum."
Then hold back of head with
hands, palms no longer on ears.
Bend trunk forward slowly
three times, each time until body
is double.

When "beating the heavenly
drum," turn body to left, then
around on right, and then to left
again, all in three reps. When
bending double, clench teeth and
breathe naturally in fine whiffs.

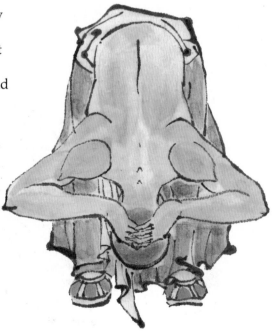

Form 12
Shake Head and Wag Tail

Continuing from last form, stretch arms sideways and frontways, where fingers are interlocked and arms bent at elbow. Turn palms downward with an internal rotation of arms. Then, with waist and belly relaxed, legs straightened and palms placed on floor, turn head and trunk to right and left. As you raise trunk to stand upright, turn palms upward with an external rotation of arms and extend them in front of chest. Bend and unbend trunk forward two times more to shake head and "wag tail" with palms on floor (left).

Closing Form: Move palms outward, toward waist sides and forward in 3 – 5 circles, fingers spread out (middle). Join palms in front of chest and move them down to lower elixir field and then to waist sides to resume starting position, with body completely relaxed and respiration naturally regulated (right).

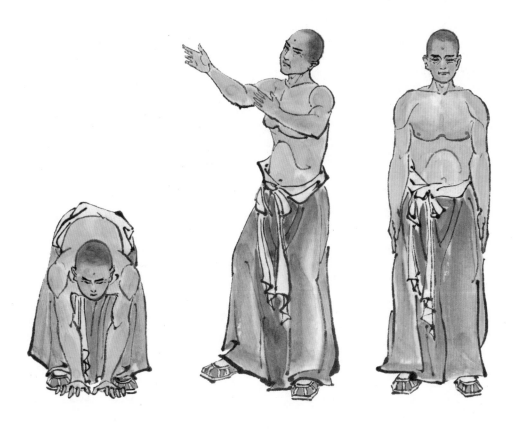

(29) The Fairies' Exercises

The following 36 exercises are selected from among a series of 47 printed in *Yi Men Guang Du*, an encyclopedia compiled by Zhou Lüjing at the turn of the 17th century.

Each form of the Fairies' Exercises has a title, describing some anecdote of a historical or legendary figure. Form 2, for example, tells about a general in the second century B.C. helping an old man put on his shoes. Considering that the anecdotes have little to do with the exercises, the title heroes are not mentioned in the English text.

Form 1
Chasing a Flying Horse

Stand with feet wider than shoulders apart, left heel raised to form a "T-step." Stretch right arm in front and left arm at back at shoulder level, as if you were holding a belt of cloth across chest. With head turned slightly to right, take nine deep breaths to conduct *qi* into left part of body. Repeat these movements, reversing right and left.

As a cure for dysentery, especially diarrhea with blood and mucus.

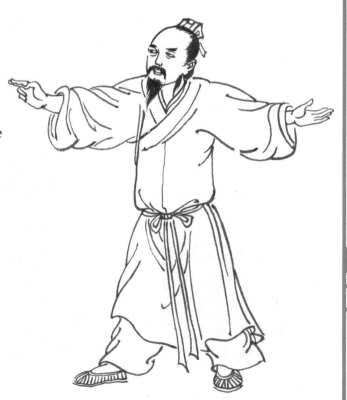

Form 2
Receiving Help
When Putting on Shoes

Sit with legs stretched in front,
feet shoulder-width apart. Press
bends of legs with both hands,
mind concentrated on the former.
Take 12 deep breaths.

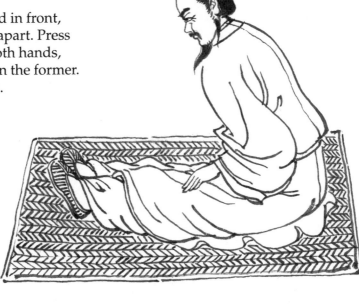

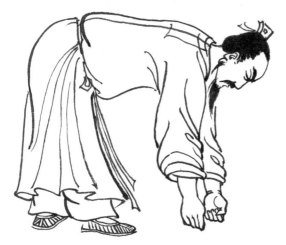

Form 3
Looking into the Well

Stand with feet apart and bend
forward until fists touch floor,
conducting *qi* into lower part of
body. Straighten body and raise
fists overhead. Breathe out
through nose in three or four
gentle whiffs.

For aching back and legs.

Form 4
Sleeping on a Rock

When on the point of seminal emission, block right nostril with a finger of left hand and press right hand on coccyx. Take deep breaths and the trouble will be over.

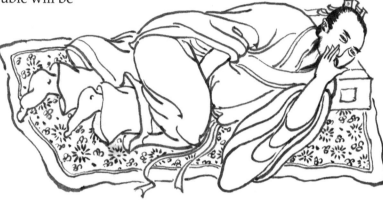

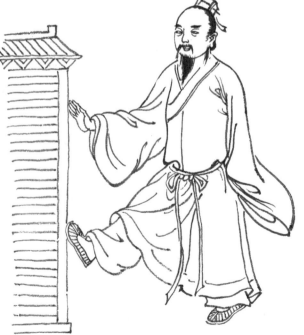

Form 5
Singing with Abandon

Stand in front of a wall, with right palm and right sole on it and left hand hanging naturally at side. Take 18 deep breaths to conduct *qi* into right part of body. Repeat these movements, reversing right and left.

For aching back.

Form 6
Fishing on Lakeside

Sit upright with legs crossed, left
fist at waist side and right hand
on right knee. Take six breaths to
conduct *qi* to affected parts.
Repeat this by reversing right and
left.

     For stubborn boils.

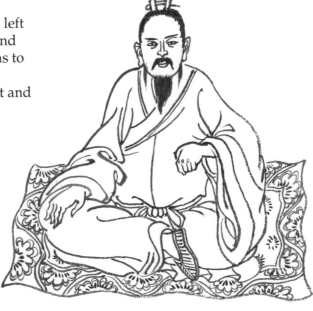

Form 7
Meditating in the
Sacred Valley

Sit upright and, with teeth
clenched, hold breath as you
place hands on back of head and
beat the heavenly drum 18 times
with fingers. (Refer to Form 11 on
p. 180.) Strike upper and lower
teeth 36 times.

     For dizziness.

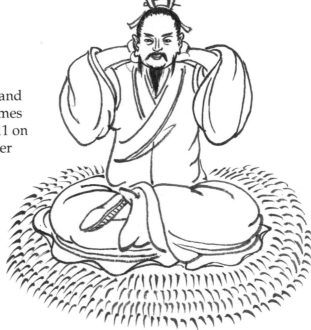

Form 8
Wrapping Up a Turban

Sit upright and hold back of head with both hands as you take 12 deep breaths.

For headache caused by the attack of pathogenic wind. (See footnote on p. 8.)

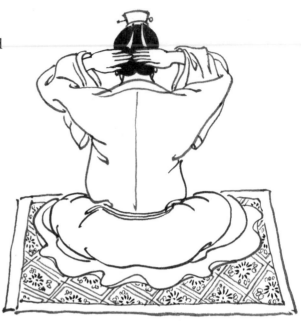

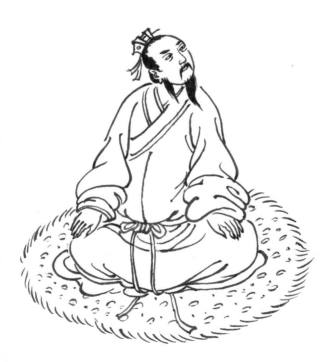

Form 9
Playing the Lute

Sit with legs crossed and palms on knees. Turn head and trunk to left and right 12 times, each accompanied by a deep breath. This is also called "Shaking the Heavenly Pillar."

For headache caused by attack of pathogenic wind and sluggishness of blood circulation.

Form 10
Lying on a Stone Couch

Lie on left side with legs bent and feet relaxed. Rub both palms until warm and hold penis and scrotum with left hand as you take 24 deep breaths to conduct *qi* into private parts.

    For diseases caused by attack of pathogenic cold.

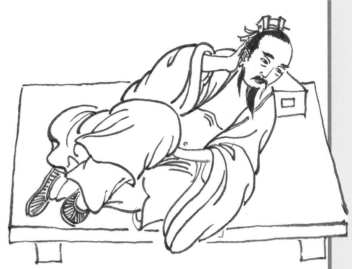

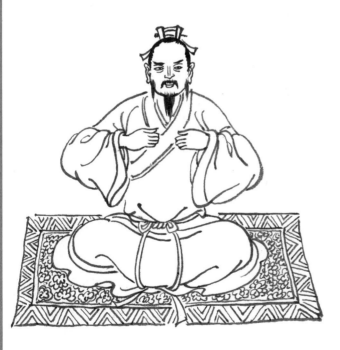

Form 11
Playing the Reed
Pipe Wind Instrument

Sit with legs crossed, arms bent at elbows and hands loosely clenched. Bend and unbend fingers nine times in front of chest, each accompanied by a deep breath to conduct *qi* into lower elixir field.

    To promote circulation of *qi* through *Ren* channel (see footnote on p. 131). For the treatment of various ailments.

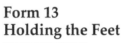

Form 12
Massaging the Kidneys

Sit with legs crossed. Rub hands until warm and massage lower back as you take 24 deep breaths to conduct *qi* into kidneys.

For kidney deficiency due to pathogenic cold and for aching back and legs.

Form 13
Holding the Feet

Sit with legs stretched in front. Hold both soles with hands as you take nine deep breaths to conduct *qi* into lower elixir field.

To stop seminal emission.

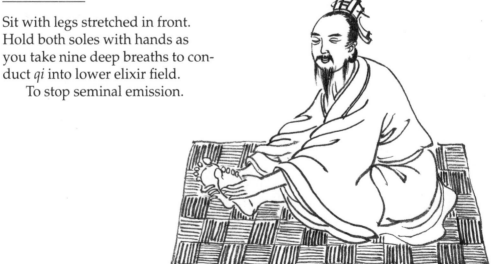

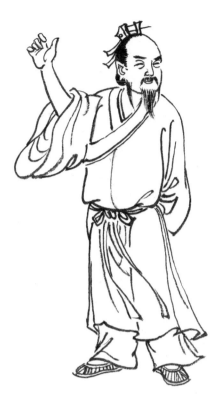

Form 14
Killing the Evil
Spirit with a Sword

Stand with feet apart, right heel
raised to form a "T-step." Raise
right hand, move left hand
behind back and turn trunk to
left, eyes looking in same
direction. Take nine deep breaths
to conduct *qi* into lower elixir
field.

    For heartache.

Form 15
Preaching Taoism

Sit on a stool with right foot on
floor and left foot off floor. Raise
left hand sideways to shoulder
level, fingers pointing up, while
right hand massages belly as you
take 12 deep breaths to conduct *qi*
into abdomen.

    For pains in back and chest.

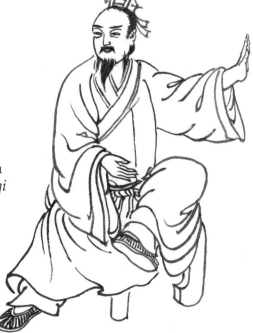

Form 16
Playing the Lute
with Hair Draped
over Shoulders

Sit upright and rub one
sole after another until
they are hot. Place palms
on knees as you take nine
deep breaths, blowing out
air through wide-open
mouth.

To promote blood cir-
culation, keep triple warmers (see footnote on p. 25)
in balance, improve weak
constitution and cure dim
eyesight.

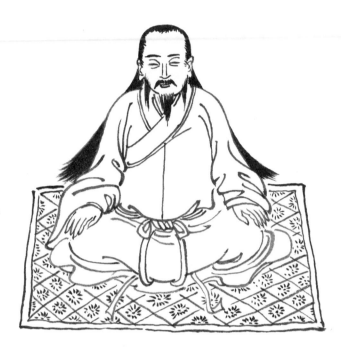

Form 17
Making a Deep Bow

Stand with feet shoulder-
width apart. Bend forward
until both palms are on
insteps. Take 24 deep
breaths. This is also called
"Black Dragon Wagging
Its Tail."

For aching back.

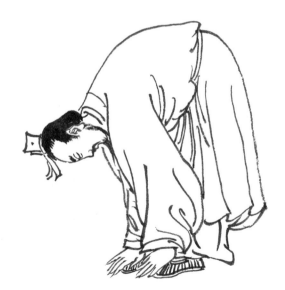

Form 18
Meditation with Eyes Closed

Sit with legs crossed and hands held together under navel. Meditate with eyes closed as you take 49 deep breaths to conduct *qi* into lower elixir field.

For abdominal pains.

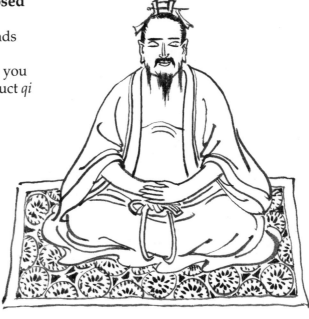

Form 19
Riding a Dragon

Sit with legs crossed and hands loosely clenched. Turn head to right as you swing up left arm and then right arm to left side. Take nine deep breaths. Repeat this by reversing right and left.

For distension and fullness in stomach and diaphragm.

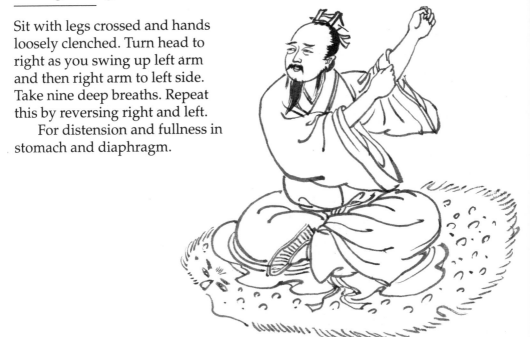

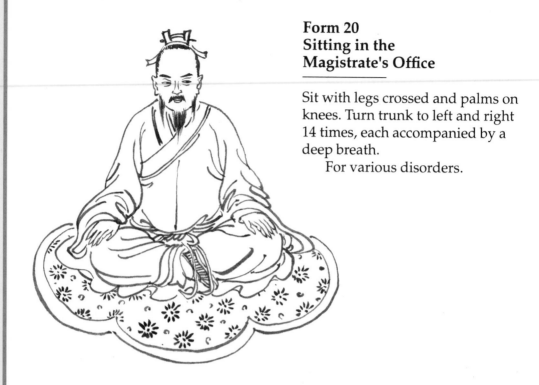

Form 20
Sitting in the
Magistrate's Office

Sit with legs crossed and palms on knees. Turn trunk to left and right 14 times, each accompanied by a deep breath.

　　For various disorders.

Form 21
Lying on the Snowy Ground

Lie on back, with legs bent or stretched out comfortably and toes turned outward. Take six deep breaths to conduct *qi* into lower elixir field as you massage chest and belly up and down, imagining that a storm is raging inside.

　　For indigestion.

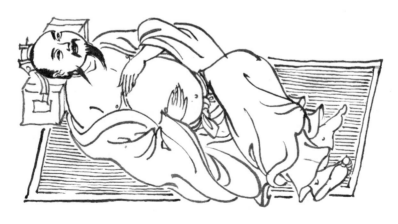

Form 22
Falling into a
Stream in Drunkenness

Lie on belly and raise head and
limbs as you take 12 deep breaths
to conduct *qi* into lower elixir
field.

    For dry cholera.

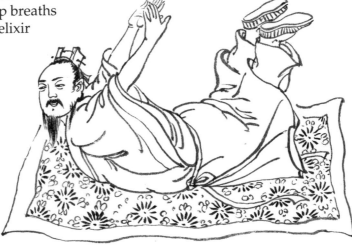

Form 23
Reaching a State
of Nothingness

Sit upright. Rub two thumbs
against middle part of right sole
as you take 24 deep breaths. Do
the same with soles alternated.

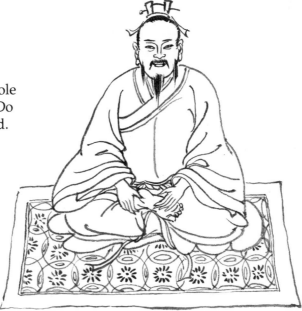

Form 24
Polishing a Mirror

Sit upright with legs
stretched in front, feet
shoulder-width apart and
toes pointing up. Raise
loosely clenched hands
frontways to shoulder
level, thumb-side up and
trunk leaning forward.
Take 12 deep breaths.

For aching all over
body.

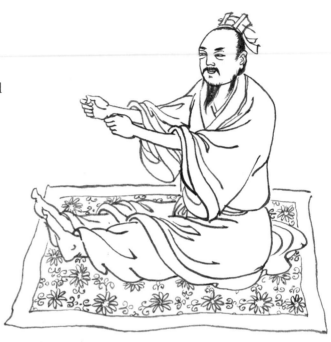

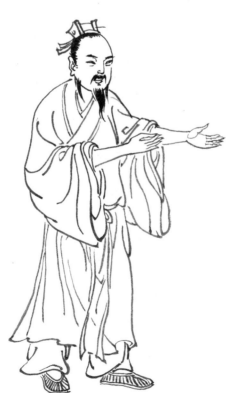

Form 25
Conducting *Qi*
through Respiration

Stand with feet shoulder-
width apart. Stretch left arm
frontways and hold inside of
forearm with right hand as
you take 22 deep breaths. Do
the same with hands
alternated.

For aching back and arms.

Form 26
Seeking a Lost Dog in Hills

Stand with left foot in front. With
forefinger of left hand pointing
forward and right hand placed at
waist side, turn head to look to
right and take 24 deep breaths to
conduct *qi* into lower elixir field.
Do the same by reversing right
and left.

For hemiparalysis.

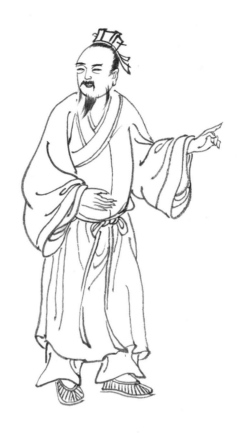

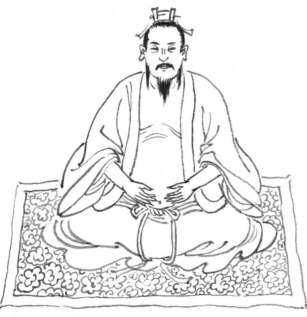

Form 27
Floating on Clouds
in an Ascent to Heaven

Sit with legs crossed. Massage
lower elixir field as you take
49 deep breaths.

For pains in small
intestines caused by attack of
pathogenic cold.

Form 28
Pinning a Flower in Hair

Sit with legs crossed. Hold back of head with both hands as you take 17 deep breaths to conduct *qi* into lower elixir field.

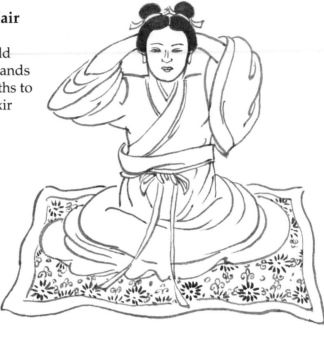

Form 29
Holding a Plank

Sit on a stool with right leg stretched to right front and left foot off floor. Turn head to right and move folded arms to left. Take 24 breaths to conduct *qi* into lower elixir field. Do the same by reversing right and left.

   For paralysis.

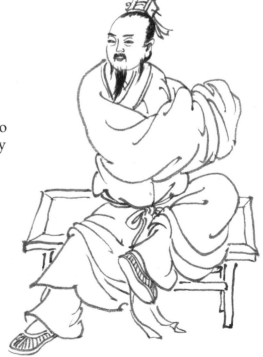

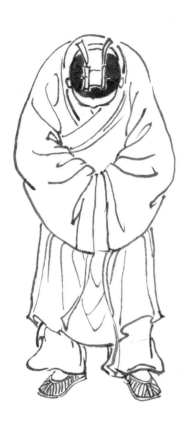

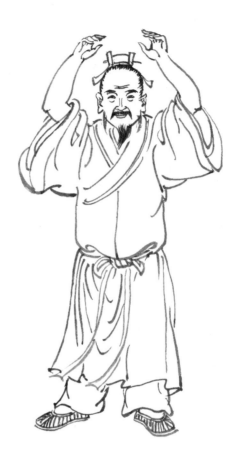

Form 30
Bowing to Heaven

Stand with feet shoulder-width
apart and toes turned outward.
Bend forward and lower head,
with hands joined in front of lower
belly. Take 17 deep breaths.

    For heartache.

Form 31
Pinning Flowers on Head

Stand with feet shoulder-width
apart and toes turned outward.
With hands raised overhead, feet
firmly purchasing ground and
anus contracted, take nine deep
breaths to conduct *qi* into lower
elixir field.

    For abdominal distension and
aching all over body.

Form 32
Playing with the
Fabled Toad in the Moon

Stand with arms akimbo, hands
clenched. Take a step forward
with left foot, body weight
equally on legs. Take 12 deep
breaths. Change feet and repeat.

For aching all over body and
febrile diseases.

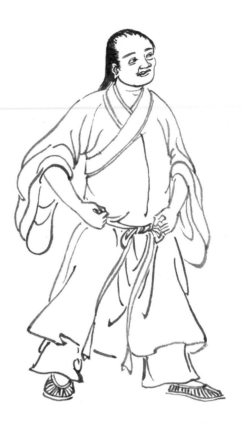

Form 33
Conducting *Qi*
through Respiration

Sit with left foot on right leg.
Place right hand on left
shoulder and left hand on
right shoulder, head turned
to look to left. Take 12 deep
breaths to conduct *qi* into
lower elixir field.

For distension and fullness
in stomach and abdomen.

Form 34
Singing Ballads in the Town

Stand with feet shoulder-width apart, taking deep breaths with right arm raised frontways at shoulder level and left hand placed above navel to quicken flow of blood and *qi* in right part of body. Do the same with hands alternated to benefit left part of body.

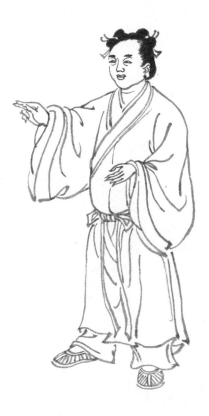

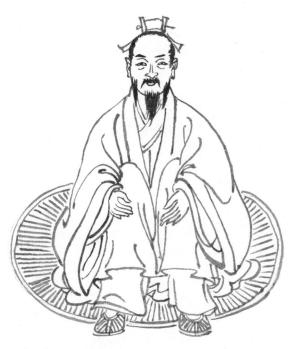

Form 35
Sitting in a Leisurely Mood

Sit with knees bent in front of belly. Massage waist sides with hands several times. Sit with both hands holding knees as you take 32 deep breaths to conduct *qi* into affected parts.

Form 36
Concluding Form

Stand at ease with body relaxed,
imagining yourself as a fairy
living a plain life and wandering
happily among the clouds.

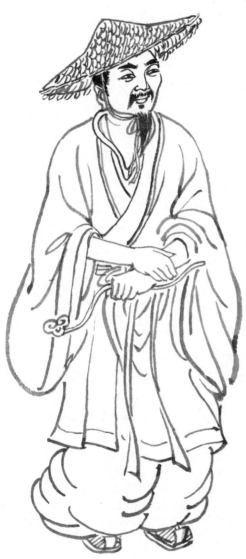

(30) Chen Huashan's Lying Exercises in Twelve Forms

Chen Huashan, a Taoist in the Northern Song Dynasty (960 – 1127), derived his name from Mount Huashan where he spent years in transcendental meditation and became a fairy. His lying exercises are included in *Yi Men Guang Du* (see introductory note on p. 78). All the 12 forms except Form 3 show the same body position — lying on right side, head cupped in right hand and resting on something like a pillow, left hand on left thigh and right foot tucked under left calf, eyes closed and mind absorbed in meditation. (Note the one four-color drawing in Form 3, "Harmonizing Vital Energy.")

Each form has a title telling about a Taoist engaged in some action, which conveys some philosophical idea of Taoism. According to Chinese thinkers, all phenomena in the universe are governed by the fundamental law of contradictions between *yin* and *yang*, the former meaning "negative" or "feminine" and the latter "positive" or "masculine." They also held that the universe is made of "five elements," namely, wood, fire, earth, metal, and water, which supplement and repel one another. These theories are widely applied in traditional Chinese medicine in expounding a physiopathological relationship among the internal organs and the unity of the universe and human body, which constitutes the three essentials of *jing* (essence), *qi* (vital energy) and *shen* (spirit or mentality).

The different titles for Huashan's lying exercises suggest that though identical in body position, practitioners may attain different frames of mind in transcendental meditation. What is required of a beginner is to lie as instructed and, with all stray thoughts banished from the mind, to reach a serene mood that will be of great benefit to the physique and mentality.

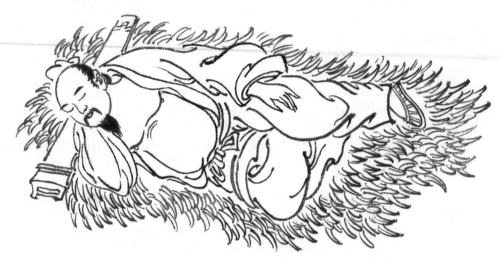

Form 1
Mao Xuanhan Subdues the Dragon and Tiger

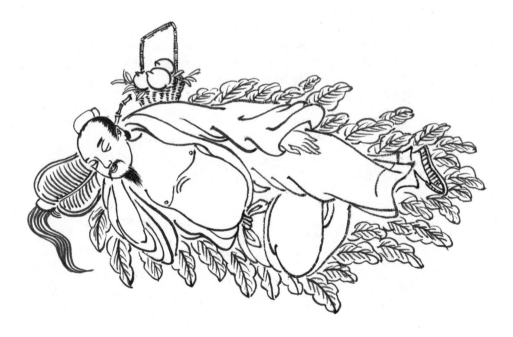

Form 2
Qu Shangpu Tempers His Soul

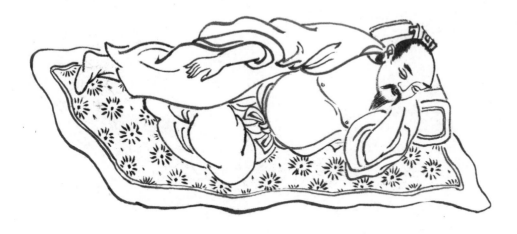

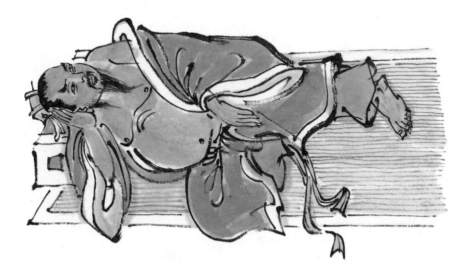

Form 3
Rev. Mayi Harmonizes Vital Energy

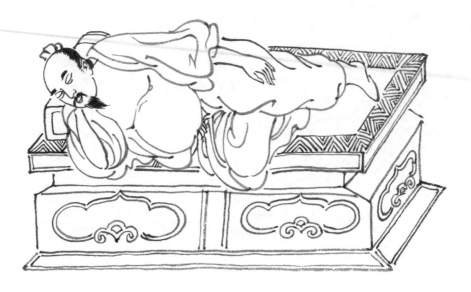

Form 4
Hu Donglin Transmits *Yin* and *Yang*

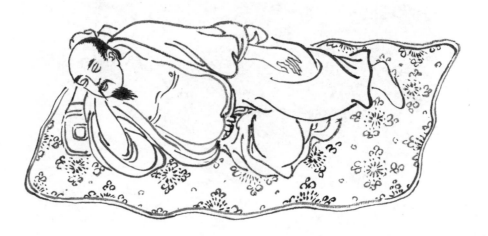

Form 5
Du Shengzhen Keeps *Yin* and *Yang* in Equilibrium

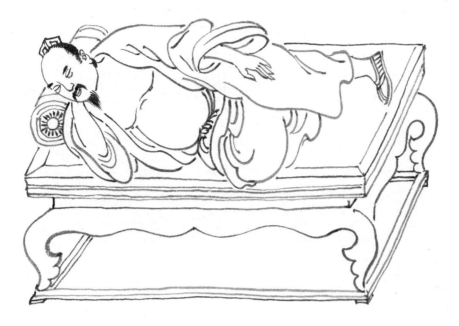

Form 6
Wang Longtu Cultivates the Fire

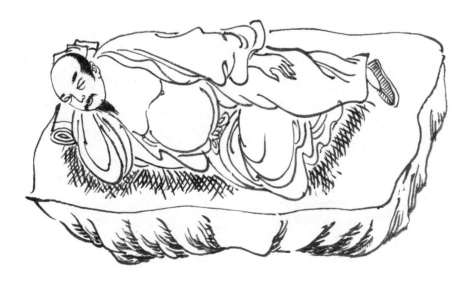

Form 7
Kang Nanyan Watches the Furnace for Making Tripods

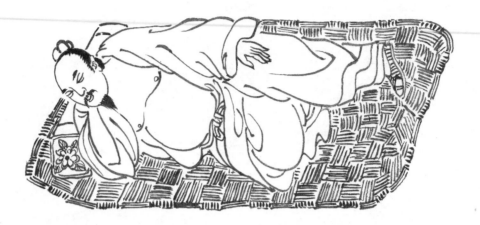

Form 8
Zhang Yitang Reserves Essence in Body

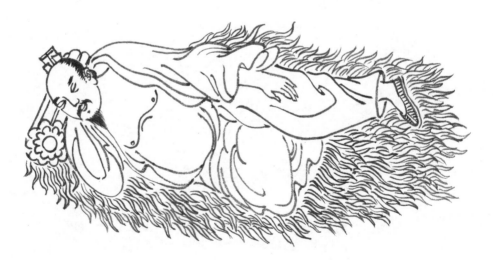

Form 9
**Zhang Xuanxuan Rests Calmly with
the Horses and Monkeys Tethered**

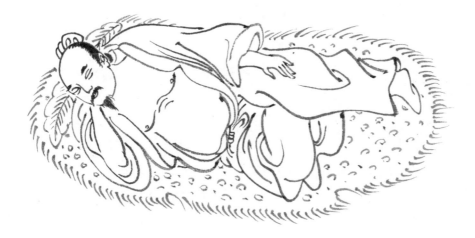

Form 10
Peng Lanweng Searches for Elixir

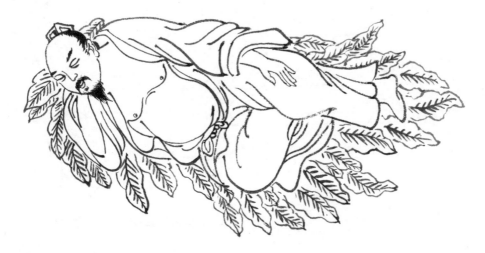

Form 11
Tang Ziran Awakens to Truth

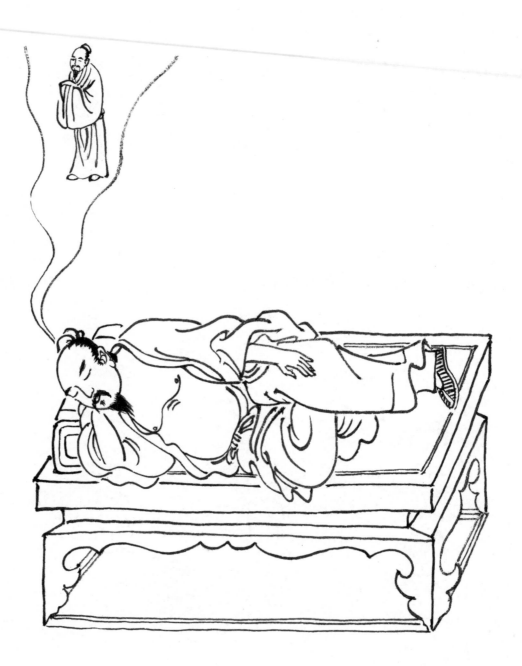

Form 12
Yu Yiyang Gains Immortality

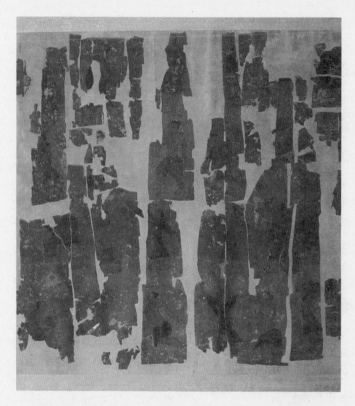

Illustration 2

Daoyin exercises painted on a piece of
silk unearthed from a tomb of the
Western Han Dynasty (206 B.C.–A.D. 24).

Glossary

akimbo – hands on hips, elbows out

aphtha – blisters in mouth; thrush

apoplexy – sudden loss of muscular control, sensation, or awareness, caused by stroke or blockage of artery to the brain. *Hemiapoplexy* affects only one side of body.

ardor urine – a burning feeling during urination

axilla – armpit

borborygmus – rumbling sound of gas passing through intestine

canthus – corner of the eye where the eyelids meet

chi – see *qi*

Chi Gung – see *Qi Gong*

chilblain – frostbite; swelling and/or itching in feet, toes, or fingers

cholera – an intestinal disease often accompanied by diarrhea, vomiting, and dehydration

consumptive diseases – tubercular afflictions

cudgel – short, heavy club

daoyin – to conduct, to guide, induce

dacryorrhea – flowing tears

dementia – madness, insanity

dermic pain – skin pain

dipsesis – great thirst

distension – expanded, blown up, stretched out

dorsal flexion – bending backward

dyspnea – shortness of breath

dysuria – painful urination

edema – swelling

elixir fields – *lower elixir field* is upper two thirds of line joining navel and pubic bone; *middle elixir field* is lower part of sternum; *upper elixir field* is between the eyebrows, just above the nose

enuresis – uncontrolled urination

facial hemiparalysis – paralysis of one side of face

fairy – immortal

febrile diseases – feverish diseases

gingival atrophy – receding gums

glabella – part of forehead above line of eyebrows, directly above root of nose

heartache – grief; anguish of mind; sorrow

hemiplegia – paralysis on one side of body

hemoptysis – spitting blood

hypochondrium – upper lateral portion of abdomen below lower ribs

inguinal hernia – hernia in area of groin

jingluo channels – network of passages through which qi (vital energy) circulates and along which acupuncture points are distributed. By means of jingluo, the ten fingers are connected with the cranial nerve and vital organs.

lumbus – lower back between hip bones and ribs; the loin

nodulation – swelling; formation of nodes

oliguria – less urination

paravertebral musculature – muscles along spine

pathogenic – causing disease

pathogenic factors – wind, cold, dampness, mist, improper diet; also called pathogens

pharyngalgia – throat pain

pharynx – throat; passageway for air from nose to larynx and food from mouth to esophagus

photophobia – sensitivity to light; often caused by measles or other conditions

physiopathological – referring to functional changes associated with or resulting from disease or injury

piles – hemorrhoids

polyorexia – overeating

preauricular heat – heat in front of ear

precordial pain – pain near the heart

proctoptosis – when anus and rectum slip out of place

pronate – to rotate palm down or backward

purchasing – gripping

qi (also *chi* or *ch'i*) – vital breath; energy which animates the cosmos; the life force energy distributed through invisible channels in the human body

Qi Gong (also *Chi Gung* or *Chi Gong*) – traditional Chinese internal energy exercises that work on balancing or strengthening qi

ren channel (also *front midline channel*) – passageway from pelvic cavity up to eyes along which qi flows

reps – repetitions

retroauricular pains – pains behind ear

scabies – contagious, itchy skin disease caused by a parasite

sputum – saliva; spit

superimpose (palms) – to place (palms); lay over or above something

supinate – to rotate palm up or forward

supraclavicular fossa – collarbones

symphysis pubis – bony structure under pubic hair; where pubic bones meet at midline of lower part of abdomen

Tao (pronounced *"dow"*) – usually translated as "the way" but no English word is equivalent. The interaction of yin and yang. Everything that serves the true nature of life is Tao.

tinnitus – ringing in the ear caused by internal defect

triple warmers (upper, middle, lower) – warmers housing some of the internal organs and functioning as passageway of qi and fluids

umbilicus – navel or "belly button"

urethrophraxis – blockage in urethra

xiphoid process – sword-shaped lowest portion of sternum

About the Authors

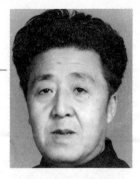

Zong Wu

Zong Wu (real name Yang Yashan) was born in 1927, is editor emeritus of *Sports Review* magazine, and is on the China National Martial Arts Committee. He is a member of the China Sports History Society and the Beijing Sports History Society and an advisor to the Henan Shaolin Temple Martial Arts Committee.

Li Mao (real name Li Shixin) was born in 1941 and started studying martial arts at age 7. He graduated from Beijing Sports Academy in 1961 and from the Academy's Martial Arts Department in 1965. He is currently a professor at Beijing University's Martial Arts Department and head of Beijing University's Martial Arts Qi Gong Society. He has written over 30 books on martial arts, including *Concise Martial Arts Dictionary, Illustrated Methods of Qi Gong, Shaolin 18 Lohan Fists, Secrets of Karate* and *Ancient Chinese Health Cookbook.*

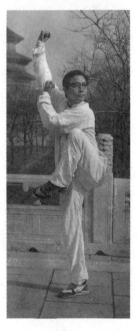

Li Mao

CREDITS
Editor, Original English Edition: Liu Yuxian
Editors, American Edition: Lloyd Kahn • Marianne Rogoff
Graphic Design: Becky Leung Yuk Shan
Graphic Design, American Edition: David Wills
Typesetting: Alphatype, Novato, California
Book Production: Janet Bollow Associates, San Anselmo, California
Typeface: Palatino (text) with Optima
Hardware: Macintosh II FX
Software: Quark Express 3.1
Color Separations: Goudy Color Separations (Scanner) Ltd., Hong Kong
Printing: Sung-In Printers, Seoul, Korea
Print Brokers: Cindy Peer, P. Chan & Edward, Inc., Mill Valley, California

These people helped make this edition possible:
Roger Carlon
Jonathan Finegold
Jane Hallander
Hal Hershey
Stephen Horowitz
Stuart Kenter
Irene Li Yuet Mei
Shao Thorpe
Qian Wangsi

FURTHER READING

For a catalog of books on Chi Gung, Tai Chi and other martial arts, write:

Eastwind Books and Arts Inc
1435 A Stockton Street
San Francisco CA 94133
(415) 772-5899

For a catalog of other Shelter fitness books, write:

Shelter Publications Inc
PO Box 279
Bolinas CA 94924
(415) 868-0280